Introduction to Oral Immunology

Introduction to Oral Immunology

A. E. Dolby

Professor, Department of Periodontology, Dental School, Welsh National School of Medicine

D. M. Walker

Senior Lecturer, Department of Oral Medicine and Oral Pathology, Dental School
Welsh National School of Medicine

N. Matthews

Senior Lecturer, Department of Medical Microbiology
Welsh National School of Medicine

W. B. Saunders Company

First published 1981
by Edward Arnold (Publishers) Ltd.
41 Bedford Square, London WC1B 3DQ

Distributed in the United States by W. B. Saunders Company,
West Washington Square, Philadelphia, PA 19105.

ISBN 0-7216-3130-4
Library of Congress Catalog Card Number 81-48637

Printed in Great Britain

Preface

It was felt that there is a need for a small introductory text dealing with the special aspects of dental and oral immunology. It has been assumed that the student would have attended a course in basic immunology before using this book, although the essential concepts of this discipline have been revised at relevant points in the text.

A detailed picture is available in some areas of oral immunology, for example the structure and function of secretory IgA in saliva, because secretory immunoglobulin from this source was the subject of many early studies as a model of this type of molecule. Conversely, research into neoplasms of the mouth has lagged behind that of tumours arising at other sites. Consequently, some concepts of immune mechanisms involved in oral cancer are necessarily extrapolations derived from our general knowledge of immunity and neoplasia.

The subject has expanded rapidly; in producing a short introduction there has been an inevitable risk of over-simplification. Again, it has been difficult to derive general principles from recent, often conflicting, research. Despite these hazards, the authors felt that it was important to keep the volume small and to make statements to which the student could later add the provisos.

We are grateful to Professor B. Cohen, Department of Dental Science, Royal College of Surgeons of England, for his helpful advice and criticism during the preparation of the manuscript. We would like to thank Mrs V.Davis and Mrs O.Hancock for their secretarial assistance and the artists for their graphical work.

Cardiff, 1981
AED
DMW
NM

Contents

1

Host Defence Components of the Mouth

Innate immunity: non-specific defence mechanisms

Host defences against infection can be divided into two categories, (a) specific and (b) non-specific immunity. The specific mechanisms usually require previous exposure to a particular micro-organism and the response is restricted to that organism. In contrast, the non-specific mechanisms do not require previous exposure and are effective against many different micro-organisms. Immunity may be purely genetically determined (innate) although other factors are often involved, as shown in the following examples.

Caries and periodontal disease vary in severity in different species. In both diseases infective agents are involved and the species variation could be accounted for by differences in innate immunity. However, diet is an overriding aetiological factor and the species variation could equally well be explained by differences in diet. Indeed beagle dogs, which are not prone to periodontal disease, can develop the disorder if fed an unnatural diet and dental caries occurs in monkeys given a sucrose-rich diet, although these animals are caries free when living in the wild.

In humans, difference in disease susceptibility between races may be genetically related, although again other factors such as diet complicate the issue. An extreme illustration of this is the increased susceptibility to infection associated with malnutrition. For example, in undernourished individuals, acute ulcerative gingivitis often progresses to cancrum oris.

Normal anatomical barriers
Mucosa
The intact oral mucosa is a barrier against infecting organisms. Although superficial squamous cells may be colonized with bacteria in the same way as squamous cells on the skin, effete cells pass to the stomach where the bacteria are attacked by hydrochloric acid. However, intact bacteria can cross a damaged epithelial barrier. The undamaged oral mucosa is permeable to a range of substances smaller

1

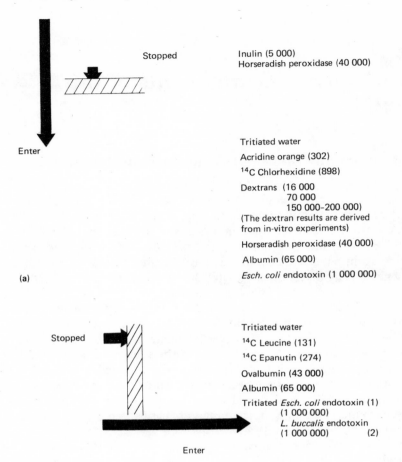

Stopped — Inulin (5 000)
Horseradish peroxidase (40 000)

Enter

Tritiated water

Acridine orange (302)

^{14}C Chlorhexidine (898)

Dextrans (16 000
70 000
150 000–200 000)
(The dextran results are derived
from in-vitro experiments)

Horseradish peroxidase (40 000)

Albumin (65 000)

Esch. coli endotoxin (1 000 000)

(a)

Stopped —

Tritiated water

^{14}C Leucine (131)

^{14}C Epanutin (274)

Ovalbumin (43 000)

Albumin (65 000)

Tritiated *Esch. coli* endotoxin (1)
(1 000 000)
L. buccalis endotoxin
(1 000 000)   (2)

Enter

1. Determined by autoradiography
2. Determined by biological effect; endotoxin can be split into
400 000 dalton units which are still biologically active

(b)

Fig. 1.1 (a) Passage of substances through oral mucosa (molecular weight).
(b) Passage of substances through gingival crevice.

than bacteria (Fig. 1.1). Several problems arise in interpreting the experimental data upon which the knowledge of the passage of materials through the oral mucosa is based.

1. Absorption through the mucosae of animals may differ from absorption through human mucosa.

2. Experiments involving general anaesthesia may alter normal clearing mechanisms such as saliva.

3. Some of the evidence is based upon examination of the mucosa which has been excised from an experimental animal and which cannot take into account the clearance of materials penetrating the mucosa by the circulating blood.

The ability of the mucosa to prevent the entry of materials is due to barriers within both the epithelium and the basement membrane (Fig. 1.2). The epithelial barrier is thought to be due to membrane-coating granules adjacent to the superficial plasma membrane of the epithelial cells. These membrane-coating granules are present within both keratinized and non-keratinized oral epithelium although the granules are morphologically dissimilar. Nonetheless, a large range of materials is capable of passing through the oral mucosa (Fig. 1.1). The barrier does not act as a simple sieve, since inulin (mol. wt. 5000) is impeded and dextran (mol. wt 20 000) is not. In addition, there is apparently a directional difference in the rate of movement of materials across the mucosa, certain materials passing faster on an outward passage than on an inward passage. The differential rates of passage may be of importance in that they determine the level at which antigen and antibody may combine within the mucosa.

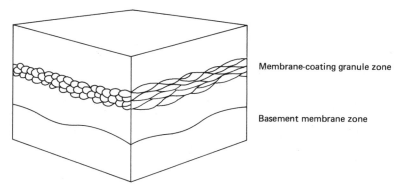

Membrane-coating granule zone

Basement membrane zone

Fig. 1.2 Barrier zones in the oral mucosa.

Gingival crevice

Since the gingival crevice may harbour micro-organisms and their products, the ability of the junctional epithelium to withstand penetration may be of considerable importance.

The junctional epithelium (Fig. 1.3) differs from the oral mucosa in several respects. The junctional epithelium is apparently more permeable than other non-keratinized oral mucosa. In addition, the

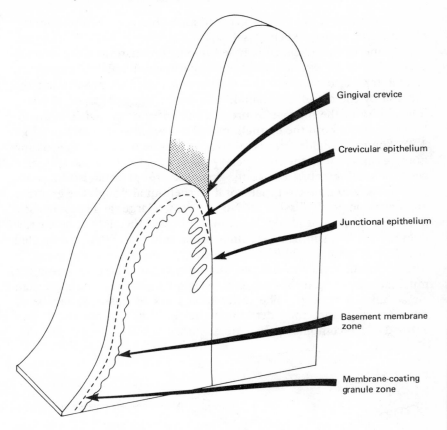

Gingival crevice

Crevicular epithelium

Junctional epithelium

Basement membrane zone

Membrane-coating granule zone

Fig. 1.3   The gingival crevice area and barriers.

epithelial cells of the junctional epithelium are capable of pinocytosing material passing through the epithelium and are reminiscent of the cuboidal cells of the Peyer's patches of the small intestine. The latter are thought to be of importance in sampling antigen presented to the small intestine, but their relationship to the Langerhans cells is not clear. In inflammation, the spaces between the epithelial cells become wider, the basal lamina decreases in width and may occasionally be absent in the deeper areas of periodontal pockets so that any barrier effect is reduced.

In health, there is a flow of fluid through the junctional epithelium into the gingival crevice. As well as exerting a flushing action, this fluid also contains blood-derived polymorphonuclear leucocytes and mononuclear phagocytes, both capable of phagocytosing bacteria.

Saliva

Saliva is a dynamic barrier in the mouth, constantly flowing backwards to the oesophagus. Micro-organisms become entrapped and are carried via the oesophagus to the hydrochloric acid and pepsin of the stomach. The gingivitis that accompanies incompetent lip posture and mouth breathing may well be explained by the loss of salivary flow. Saliva also acts as an additional barrier to the penetration of materials into the oral mucosa; in experiments where salivation has been reduced by hyoscine, penetration of various materials (acridine orange, thioflavine) has been enhanced.

Further, saliva contains a number of materials which afford non-specific protection to the individual. Thus lysozyme, a mucolytic enzyme, is capable of splitting sugars off the glycopeptides of the cell wall of many Gram-positive bacteria, leading to their lysis. Although lysozyme is detectable in gingival crevice fluid and is found in the leucocytes migrating into the mouth, the major source is the salivary glands. The organism *Micrococcus lysodeikticus* is readily lysed by lysozyme and is used as a target in assays of the enzyme. Since the origin of the enzyme is predominantly from the salivary glands, this lysozyme assay has been used as an index of salivary flow.

Other substances in saliva with antimicrobial activity include lactoferrin, which reduces the amount of free iron available for bacterial metabolism, unidentified basic polypeptides, which exert antimicrobial activity, and lactoperoxidase which can cross-link proteins and hence damage certain bacteria and viruses. The mucins of saliva have some carbohydrate side chains in common with epithelial cells and competitively inhibit the binding of viruses to the epithelial cells.

Specific defence components of the mouth

Saliva

In addition to affording non-specific protection, saliva also contains a specific immunological defence in the form of antibodies. The measurement of antibody concentrations in saliva is complicated by several factors which should be taken into account when comparing such levels in disease. Whole saliva is often contaminated by materials which modify the level of detectable antibody. For example, bacterial enzyme contamination reduces the level, whereas transudation of antibody via the gingival crevice increases the level of antibody. The levels have to be related to volume, which varies from individual to individual and may be stimulated or unstimulated. Measurement of salivary antibody produced by the parotid gland with cannulation of

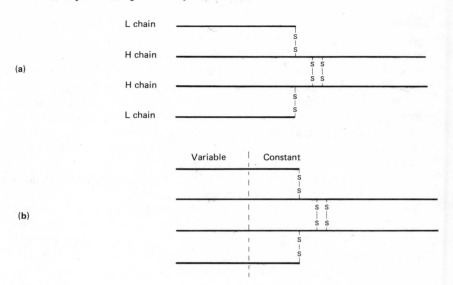

Fig. 1.4 Diagrammatic representation of antibody structure. **(a)** Structure showing two short (L = light) and two long (H = heavy) polypeptide chains held together by disulphide bridges (-s-s-). For any given antibody molecule the amino acid sequences of the two L chains are identical to one another; similarly, the two H chains have identical sequences. **(b)** Comparison of the amino acid sequences of different antibody molecules has revealed major differences in the so-called variable region—comprising approximately half of the L chain and a quarter of the H chains. **(c)** The antigen-binding sites are in the variable region. Only some of the amino acid residues of the variable region are involved—three separate stretches

the duct overcomes the problem of contamination but gives a measurement related to parotid saliva alone. Comparison of antibody levels in saliva and serum reveals several differences both in concentration and type of antibody. A proportion of the antibody in the saliva is derived from the blood flowing through the salivary gland, although most is synthesized by plasma cells within the gland and is actively transported. The major immunoglobulin of saliva and other digestive juices as well as respiratory secretions and most external secretions is IgA. Salivary IgA differs from serum IgA in several respects. Secretory IgA is a dimer (mol. wt 390 000) made up of two subunits, each the size of the serum IgA monomer (mol. wt. 160 000), plus secretory component (mol. wt. 58 000) and J-chain (mol. wt. 15 000). The diagrammatic representation of antibody structure is shown in Fig. 1.4. Comparison of secretory IgA with IgG is shown in Fig. 1.5

Each IgA monomer is linked by two disulphide bridges to the J chain, which is probably responsible for maintaining the dimeric

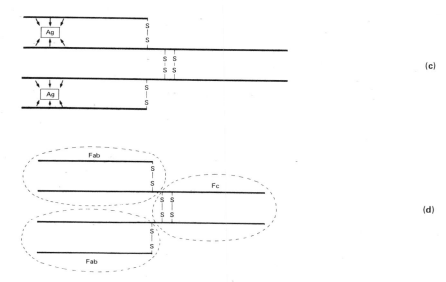

(c)

(d)

within the L chain and three within the H chain. As each antigen-binding site involves H and L chain sequences, there are two antigen-binding sites per molecule. **(d)** The original studies on antibody structure employed proteolytic enzyme degradation. Under suitable conditions, the H chain can be cleaved to produce two Fab fragments (Fab = fragment antigen binding) and one Fc fragment (Fc = fragment crystallizable). NB Different antibody classes are distinguishable by differences in amino acid sequences within the constant region of the heavy chain. Further, although IgG, IgD and IgE have structures approximating to the above, IgM is a pentamer of the basic structure and secretory IgA is a dimer (see Fig. 1.5).

structure, for the binding of secretory component and is also a plasma cell product. Secretory component is produced by epithelial cells within the salivary gland and it is important in transport of the IgA across the salivary duct epithelium. It also serves to stabilize the molecule against proteolytic digestion. Secretory IgA antibodies appear to be important in two ways.

Firstly, secretory IgA probably exerts its effect by preventing attachment of bacteria and viruses to the teeth and oral mucosa. Whether secretory IgA is capable of opsonizing bacteria for phagocytosis directly remains controversial; there is some evidence that complement is activated via the alternative pathway and phagocytosis may be enhanced in this way. Antibody titres of secretory IgA correlate better than serum immunoglobulins with resistance to infection by a number of viruses such as echovirus, adenovirus and coxsackie virus.

Secondly, secretory IgA antibodies are directed also against some food antigens and may represent a mechanism for protecting the

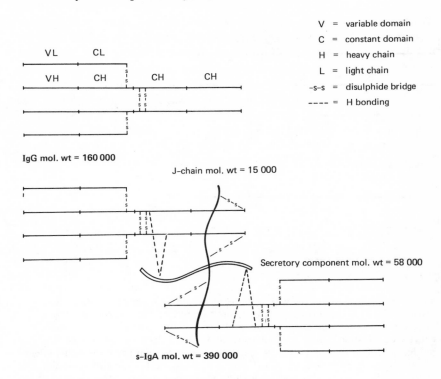

Fig. 1.5   Comparative diagrams of IgG and secretory IgA.

animal against immunological injury. A small proportion of food antigens escapes complete proteolytic digestion in the gut and antigenic material may be absorbed, so provoking an immune reaction. Several types of immune reactions may be damaging to the host, although the interaction of secretory IgA and antigen does not appear to lead to such damage. Intestinal absorption of antigen in experimental animals has been decreased by prior parenteral immunization with the corresponding antigen and the diminution may be mediated by secretory IgA. This would protect the organism against harmful antigens by forming unabsorbable complexes which would be degraded by proteolytic enzymes on the surface of the intestine. A reduction in secretory IgA is frequently accompanied by an increased tendency to allergy to antigens of food.

Gingival crevice fluid
The analysis of gingival crevice fluid presents problems similar to those listed for saliva. In addition, the amount of fluid is very small.

Since the flow of fluid is increased with gingival inflammation, more information is available about gingival crevice fluid collected in gingivitis. Capillary tubes and chromatographic paper have been used for collection, but care has to be taken that the gingival crevice has not been traumatized. Cells may also be collected from the gingival crevice area, either by imprinting them on transparent plastic for staining and enumeration, or by gently washing the area and collecting the washings for vital studies. The major immunoglobulin classes are represented in gingival crevice fluid. The concentrations of these immunoglobulins have been measured by the technique of single radial immunodiffusion.

The antiserum to a particular immunoglobulin class is incorporated in a thin layer of agar gel on a glass plate and the gingival crevice fluid is placed in small wells punched in the agar (Fig. 1.6). A precipitation ring will form around the well where the diffusing immunoglobulin is precipitated by the anti-immunoglobulin serum in the surrounding gel. The diameter squared of the ring is proportional to the concentration of the immunoglobulin in the well. From the graph of the diameter squared versus the concentration for a standard immunoglobulin preparation, the concentration of immunoglobulin in the gingival crevice fluid can be determined.

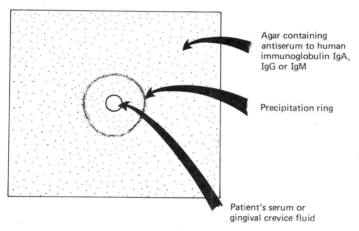

Agar containing antiserum to human immunoglobulin IgA, IgG or IgM

Precipitation ring

Patient's serum or gingival crevice fluid

Fig. 1.6 Single radial immunodiffusion.

The immunoglobulins of gingival crevice fluid represent a summation of immunoglobulin secreted by plasma cells within the gingiva plus plasma immunoglobulin passing from the blood; radiolabelled *serum* IgG and IgM have been detected in the gingival crevice fluid of experimental animals. Since secretory IgA can be distinguished from serum IgA by its secretory component, it has been possible to determine the contribution of the serum IgA to the total gingival crevice fluid IgA. The immunoglobulin levels of gingival crevice fluid are shown in Fig. 1.7.

Several components of complement (see Fig. 3.5), such as C3, C4, C5 and factor B, have been detected in gingival crevice fluid. The

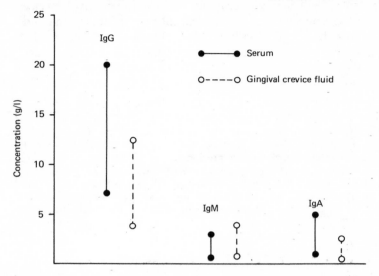

Fig. 1.7   Immunoglobulin content of serum and gingival crevice fluid compared.

concentrations of C3 and C4 are raised in the gingival crevice fluid derived from inflamed, as compared with normal, gingiva. Factor B and C5 are detectable only in the gingival crevice fluid derived from inflamed gingiva. It has been found that C3 is degraded in inflamed gingival crevice fluid, implying that complement activation is occurring within the gingival crevice.

Cellular components

The cells involved in the immune response in the mouth are widely distributed in the following sites, (1) submucosal tissue, (2) gingiva, (3) salivary glands, (4) epithelium, (5) gingival crevice fluid, (6) tonsils, and (7) extraoral lymph nodes, which drain lymph from the oral cavity (Fig. 1.8).

Submucosa; collections of lymphocytes and macrophages

These mononuclear cells are found throughout the mouth just beneath the epithelium. Unlike the Peyer's patches of the small intestine, these collections of cells are diffusely scattered and their functions are not clear.

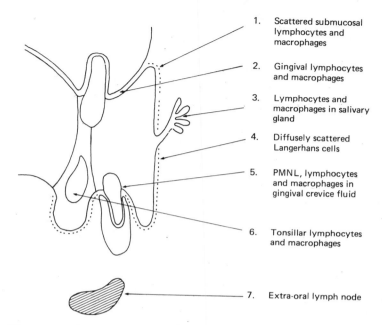

1. Scattered submucosal lymphocytes and macrophages

2. Gingival lymphocytes and macrophages

3. Lymphocytes and macrophages in salivary gland

4. Diffusely scattered Langerhans cells

5. PMNL, lymphocytes and macrophages in gingival crevice fluid

6. Tonsillar lymphocytes and macrophages

7. Extra-oral lymph node

Fig. 1.8 The major collections of lymphoid cells of the mouth.

Gingiva

An inflammatory infiltrate is invariably present in humans in healthy or diseased gingiva, and in the presence of dento-gingival plaque this is increased. Most of the plasma cells present in this infiltrate are producing IgG (Fig. 1.9). Within the junctional epithelium, small mononuclear cells termed 'inter-epithelial lymphocytes' have been found. Some lymphocytes reach the crevice; it is not known whether all inter-epithelial lymphocytes are migratory.

Salivary glands

Lymphocytes, macrophages and plasma cells are found interspersed amongst the acini of the salivary glands. Most of the plasma cells secrete IgA, although a minority secrete IgM or IgG. The epithelial cells of the ducts synthesize secretory component and it is within these cells that the dimeric IgA synthesized by adjacent plasma cells complexes to secretory component, the entire secretory IgA complex then being transmitted into the ducts (Fig. 1.10). The bulk of the IgA in saliva is of secretory type and is synthesized in the salivary glands. Information on the classes of antibody synthesized in the salivary

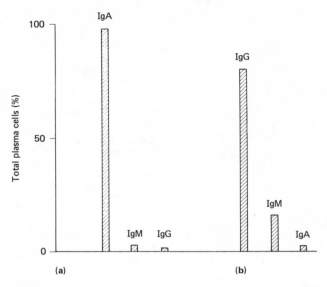

Fig. 1.9 The proportion of plasma cells producing immunoglobulin of a particular class: **(a)** in the salivary glands, and **(b)** in inflamed gingiva.

glands and their antigenic specificities has been obtained largely by the use of the techniques of immunofluorescence and plaque assay.

In immunofluorescence, the dye (fluorochrome) linked to the protein absorbs light at one wavelength and emits longer wavelength light (fluorescence), e.g. fluorescein absorbs light at 490 nm and emits it at 520 nm. Either the direct or indirect methods of fluorescent antibody labelling may be employed to identify and localize an antigen. In the direct method, the fluorochrome-labelled antibodies are brought into direct contact with the tissue section, thus allowing them to react (Fig. 1.11a). Excess antibody is washed off and the section examined with a suitable microscope—which would usually have a mercury lamp, appropriate wavelength filters and specialized objectives. The presence of antigen is indicated by a discrete area of fluorescence. In the indirect method, a non-labelled antiserum (primary antibody) is laid on first in the same way as above, but after washing, this is followed by an anti-immunoglobulin serum (secondary antibody) which is labelled with the fluorochrome (Fig. 1.11b). This indirect method is much more sensitive since each primary antibody molecule bound can be complexed by several molecules of the fluorochrome-labelled secondary antibody. In examining the salivary glands, two fluorochromes (rhodamine and fluorescein, red and green respectively) have been employed to enable the visualization of differing immuno-globulins in the same section. The use of these techniques has enabled the relative proportions of the various immunoglobulin-containing cells in the salivary glands to be determined (Fig. 1.9).

A more recent method, the plaque assay (Fig. 1.12), may be used to detect the antibody production to specific antigen rather than simply to detect immunoglobulin type. In this method the cells released *in vitro* after disruption of the gland are incubated with antigen-coated erythrocytes incorporated into a gel.

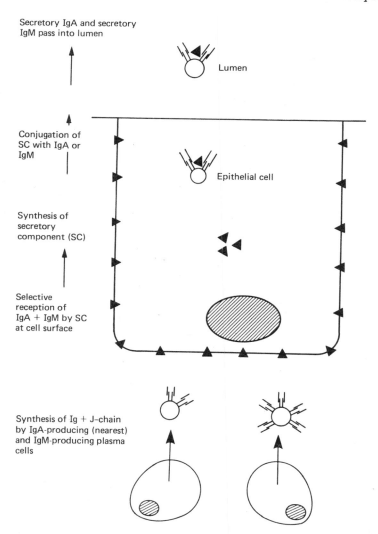

Secretory IgA and secretory
IgM pass into lumen

Lumen

Conjugation of
SC with IgA or
IgM

Epithelial cell

Synthesis of
secretory
component (SC)

Selective
reception of
IgA + IgM by SC
at cell surface

Synthesis of Ig + J–chain
by IgA-producing (nearest)
and IgM-producing plasma
cells

Fig. 1.10 Passage of secretory IgA and secretory IgM into the lumen of the salivary gland. (After a model proposed by Brandtzaeg, P. (1974). *Immunology* **26**, 1101.)

Antibody secreted by a single cell binds to adjacent antigen-coated erythrocytes. Addition of complement leads to lysis of these erythrocytes leaving a small clear zone (plaque) in the gel.

The use of this plaque assay has led to the realization that immuno-globulin-producing cells stimulated elsewhere in the gastrointestinal tract may be found in the salivary glands.

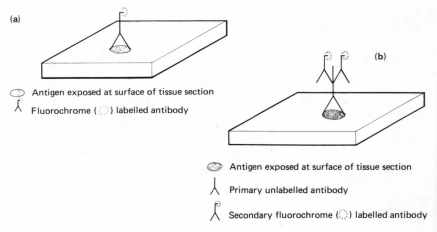

(a)

⬭ Antigen exposed at surface of tissue section

⅄ Fluorochrome ( ) labelled antibody

(b)

⬭ Antigen exposed at surface of tissue section

⅄ Primary unlabelled antibody

⅄ Secondary fluorochrome ( ) labelled antibody

Fig. 1.11   Immunofluorescent detection of tissue antigens. **(a)** Direct immunofluorescence. **(b)** Indirect immunofluorescence.

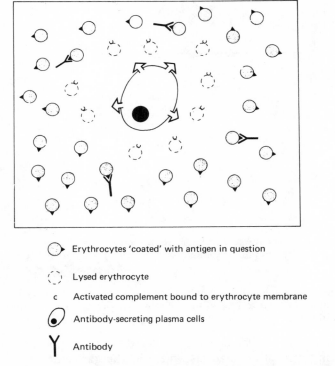

⬭ Erythrocytes 'coated' with antigen in question

⬭ Lysed erythrocyte

c   Activated complement bound to erythrocyte membrane

⬭ Antibody-secreting plasma cells

Y   Antibody

Fig. 1.12   Haemolytic plaque assay for cells secreting specific antibody.

In addition to the enumeration of immunoglobulin-forming cells by the fluorescent antibody method, the technique has also been used to determine the site of production of secretory component, the material which contributes to the passage of IgA from the lamina propria to the ducts of the gland.

Epithelium: Langerhans cells

Antigen passing through the oral mucosa is phagocytosed by Langerhans cells which are distributed above the basement membrane. They are large dendritic cells with properties akin to macrophages, i.e. mononuclear phagocytes with Fc and C3 receptors and Ia-like surface antigens (transplantation antigens found especially on B lymphocytes and macrophages and probably identical with HLA-D antigens). After phagocytosis, the Langerhans cells migrate to the local lymph node where they home to the paracortical T cell area, so initiating a cell-mediated immune response (Fig. 1.13).

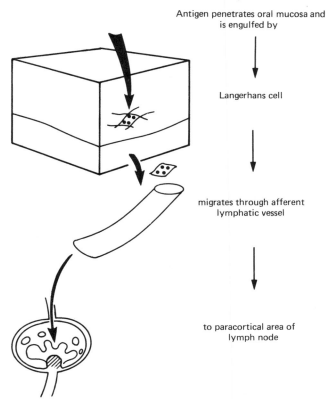

Antigen penetrates oral mucosa and is engulfed by

Langerhans cell

migrates through afferent lymphatic vessel

to paracortical area of lymph node

Fig. 1.13 Role of Langerhans cell in antigen processing in oral mucosa.

Gingival crevice fluid

The cells of the gingival crevice fluid are predominantly (90 per cent) polymorphonuclear neutrophil leucocytes (PMNL); macrophages and lymphocytes constitute approximately 10 per cent. Considerable numbers of PMNL are released into the oral cavity each minute (30 000–1 000 000). A large proportion of these cells arises from gingival crevice fluid.

About 75 per cent of the PMNL are morphologically intact and experiments in which the functions of these PMNL have been examined show that they are capable of phagocytosis and that gingival crevice fluid imparts opsonic (phagocytosis promoting) activity, presumably from the IgG and complement content. Since dental plaque has been shown to be chemotactic for PMNL, it presumably contributes to the passage of the PMNL into the gingival crevice fluid.

Tonsil and lymph node

Lymphatic channels serve to carry antigen which has entered sites throughout the oral cavity to the submental, submaxillary and deep cervical lymph nodes. The submental and submaxillary lymph nodes possess the characteristic structure of lymph nodes found elsewhere in the body (Fig. 1.14). The superficial lymphoid tissue of the intestine

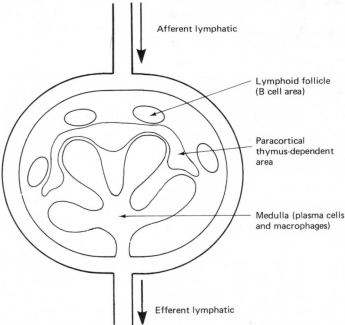

Afferent lymphatic

Lymphoid follicle (B cell area)

Paracortical thymus-dependent area

Medulla (plasma cells and macrophages)

Efferent lymphatic

Fig. 1.14 The activated lymph node.

lacks the classic dendritic reticular cells which are seen in lymph nodes and which have been associated with antigen processing and display. However, the pharyngeal, lingual and nasopharyngeal tonsil do possess dendritic reticular cells and are also sites of local antibody induction and secretion. Thus the tonsil aggregates appear to have some of the characteristics of peripheral lymph nodes, unlike the superficial lymphoid tissue of the intestine.

The lymph nodes possess functionally different areas. Depending upon the type of antigen and its presentation to the node, different types of immune response can ensue. With cell-mediated responses there is enlargement of the predominantly T lymphocyte-containing paracortical area. With antibody responses the predominantly B lymphocyte-containing cortex is involved. However, the antibody-producing plasma cells are largely found in the medulla.

The two components of the immune system

Humoral immunity

Lymphocytes arise from pluripotential stem cells in the bone marrow. During differentiation, lymphocytes can take one of two routes—to the thymus where they are processed to become T (for thymus-processed) lymphocytes or to the mammalian equivalent of the bursa of Fabricius for processing to B (for bursa-processed) lymphocytes. The bursa of Fabricius is an organ in the cloaca of birds, but the site of the mammalian equivalent is uncertain.

The role of the B lymphocyte is to differentiate into an antibody-producing plasma cell after being triggered by its specific antigen. The B lymphocyte recognizes its antigen by surface receptors, these are antibody in nature and on any particular B lymphocyte all the receptors have the same specificity, as indeed does the antibody produced by the progeny plasma cells. Some antigens can trigger the B cells by direct contact, provoking the differentiation into IgM antibody-producing cells. For the production of IgG and IgA antibody, the antigen must be presented to the B lymphocyte by macrophages and a subset of T lymphocytes known as helper T cells. In this latter case, the exact method of antigen presentation and the site of cellular co-operation is still disputed.

There are several mechanisms by which specific antibodies can combat infection. Firstly, specific antibody of any class can potentially prevent an organism attaching to a surface by masking structures on the surface of the organism, e.g. the receptors with which viruses bind to their target cell. Note how this differs from the non-specific inhibition of binding described in relation to saliva. Secondly, IgG antibodies are opsonic since phagocytic cells have receptors for the Fc tail of IgG. Thirdly, activation of complement (see Fig. 3.5) by antibodies of the IgM, IgG or IgA class can lead to opsonization via the C3b complement component. This is the mechanism which is thought to operate in the gingival crevice. Lastly, another result of complement activation may be lysis of the organism by the C8 and C9 complement components; in practice this mechanism appears to be effective against a minority of pathogenic organisms.

Cell-mediated immunity

T lymphocytes are a heterogeneous group of cells with at least three functions: (1) as helper cells in antibody production, (2) as suppressor cells damping down the antibody response, and (3) finally as effectors of cell-mediated immunity, as discussed below.

T lymphocytes constantly circulate in the blood and lymph. Like B lymphocytes, T cells have receptors for antigen. The T cell antigen receptor differs from that of the B cell in being less specific and being only part of an antibody molecule. It is a heavy chain analogue differing from the conventional type of heavy chain, but coded for by a gene adjacent to the gene responsible for the μ chain in the genome. On meeting its specific antigen, the T lymphocyte releases a family of substances termed lymphokines which act on other lymphocytes and macrophages. As a result, other lymphocytes in the vicinity are stimulated to divide and produce more lymphokines and mononuclear phagocytes are attracted to the site where they become 'activated'. Mitogenic factor, which stimulates division in lymphocytes, is the best characterized of the lymphokines acting on lymphocytes. The lymphokines acting on mononuclear phagocytes include macrophage chemotactic factor (MCF), macrophage inhibition factor (MIF) and macrophage activating factor (MAF). On activation, macrophages become more phagocytic, produce more lysosomal enzymes and are more able to kill ingested pathogens. Most lymphokines have similar physicochemical properties and it is possible that different activities of lymphokines as measured *in vitro* are due to the same substance, for example MIF and MAF may be the same molecule. *In vivo*, lymphokines may:

(i) promote phagocytosis and intracellular killing by mononuclear phagocytes;

(ii) as interferon (γ type), regulate the activity of mononuclear cells;

(iii) as lymphotoxins, produce local tissue damage.

T cells may also induce cell destruction by direct cell/cell contact without the involvement of lymphotoxin—these are termed cytotoxic T lymphocytes. In cell-mediated reactions, the cells involved are largely lymphocytes and macrophages and this is reflected in the histology where a predominantly mononuclear cell infiltrate is seen. Cell-mediated immunity is of major importance in combating viral and intracellular bacterial infections. In viral infections, cytotoxic T cells recognize not just the viral antigens on the infected cell surface, but a complex of viral antigen and transplantation antigen, i.e. modified transplantation antigen. This may explain why a tissue graft from an unrelated individual is so efficiently rejected—the transplantation antigens of the graft are seen as modified self in the same manner as virally infected cells.

The GALT system and the mouth

B and T lymphocytes recirculate from the blood to the lymph and back again. The passage from blood to lymph occurs in specialized blood vessels termed post-capillary venules, which are found in lymph nodes. From the efferent lymphatic vessel, the lymphocytes travel to the thoracic duct and then back into the bloodstream. In recent years, it has become apparent that there are at least two circulatory systems sharing the classical blood-thoracic duct route described above. One such route involves the gut-associated lymphoid tissue (GALT) which comprises the Peyer's patches, appendix and tonsils. Antigen-triggered lymphocytes from the Peyer's patches travel via the lymphatics and blood vessels to the mesenteric lymph nodes, lactating mammary gland, salivary gland and lamina propria of the gut. The migrating cells are mostly precursors of IgA-producing plasma cells but the method by which they 'home' is unknown, although use is probably made of common cell receptors. Because of the GALT route, it is possible that lymphocytes sensitized to antigen in the lower portion of the gut may 'home' to the mouth. Surprisingly, unlike antibody responses elsewhere in the body, the secretory IgA response has poor memory—repeated exposure to antigen does not result in a more rapid, increased secretory IgA response.

Summary

The defence mechanisms of the mouth are both non-specific and specific. Not all materials which may be potentially harmful will cross the mucosal barrier, those that do being met by an immune system which produces antibody to neutralize on the mucosal surface and to facilitate the phagocytosis of material within the tissue. The protective mechanism also involves the use of cells released into the mouth which appear capable of phagocytosing and killing bacteria. However, under certain circumstances the immune response may lead to the release of soluble mediators which may produce local tissue damage.

Further reading

Brandtzaeg, P. (1977). Intestinal secretion of IgA and IgM: a hypothetical model. *Ciba Foundation Symposium* **46**, 77–108.

Cimasoni, G., Ishikawa, I. and Jaccard, F. (1977). Enzyme activity in the gingival crevice. In *The Borderland between Caries and Periodontal Disease*, pp. 13–41. Ed. by T. Lehner. Academic Press, London.

Page, R. C. and Schroeder, H. E. (1976). Pathogenesis of inflammatory periodontal disease. A summary of current work. Laboratory *Investigation* **34**, 235–49.

Schroeder, H. E. (1977). Histopathology of the gingival sulcus. In *The Borderland between Caries and Periodontal Disease*, pp. 43–78. Ed. by T. Lehner. Academic Press, London.

Squier, C. A., Johnson, N. W. and Hackemann, Margarete (1975). Structure and function of normal human oral mucosa. In *Oral Mucosa in Health and Disease*, pp. 1–112. Ed. by A. E. Dolby. Blackwell Scientific, Oxford.

Wright, Ralph (1977). *Immunology of Gastrointestinal and Liver Disease*. Current Topics in Immunology Series No. 8. Ed. by John Turk. Edward Arnold, London.

2

Dental Caries, Pulpal and Periapical Conditions

Dental caries

In the initial lesion of dental caries, enamel is demineralized by acid formed from dietary sugars (particularly sucrose) by the bacteria in dental plaque (Fig. 2.1). In a progressive lesion, bacteria subsequently invade this altered enamel. Similarly, involvement of the dentine features an early phase of decalcification before invasion by the bacteria which penetrate the dentinal tubules at the advancing front of the lesion. Proteolytic bacteria digest the collagen fibres of the dentinal matrix.

Dental plaque is an aggregation of many different bacteria and their products on the tooth surface. The evidence incriminating *Streptococcus mutans* as the most important cariogenic organism is considerable.

1. When germ-free rats on a sucrose-rich diet are mono-inoculated with *Strept. mutans*, caries results. It should be noted, however, that other bacteria, *Strept. sanguis, Strept. faecalis, Lactobacillus acidophilus* and *Actinomyces viscosus* can also induce caries in such experiments.

2. *Strept. mutans* can be isolated from plaque on carious teeth and from the lesion, and is found more frequently in the plaque of caries-active subjects compared with that of caries-free subjects.

3. Patients with active caries have raised serum levels of antibody against the organism.

4. Immunization with *Strept. mutans* can prevent caries in monkeys and rats.

Formation of dental plaque
A thin amorphous film, the acquired salivary pellicle is formed on the enamel surface by selective adsorption of salivary constituents.

Strept. mutans (and other bacteria) initially adhere to this pellicle possibly by specific binding sites, which may be lectin-like (sugar-binding proteins, Fig. 2.2).

22

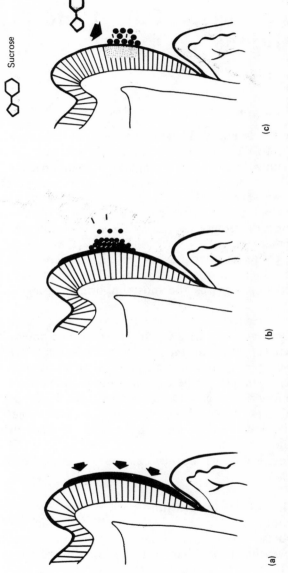

Fig. 2.1 The initiation of caries. (a) Salivary glycoproteins are deposited on enamel surfaces. (b) Bacteria colonize this acquired salivary pellicle to form plaque. (c) Dietary sucrose utilized by plaque bacteria to form acid, which demineralizes enamel. (Diagrams are not to scale).

The third stage of plaque formation involves the aggregation and cohesion of the *Strept. mutans* by the extracellular polysaccharides, in particular glucans, which the organisms themselves elaborate.

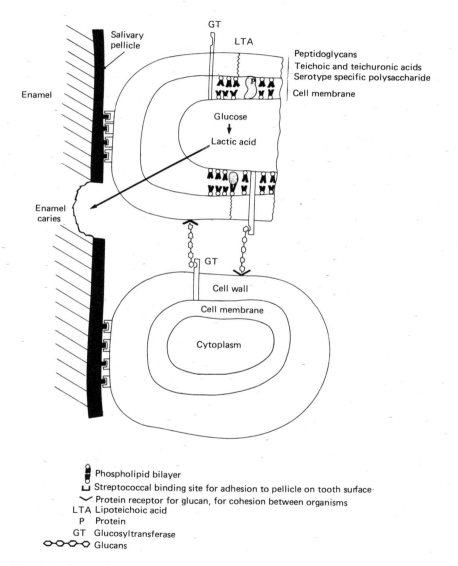

Fig. 2.2 Schematic representation of the structure of *Streptococcus mutans*.

Enzymes of *Strept. mutans* implicated in the pathogenesis of caries (Fig. 2.2)

Cariogenic strains of *Strept. mutans* have enzymes called glucosyltransferases which can synthesize large amounts of extracellular polysaccharides (glucans) from dietary sucrose using the energy of its disaccharide bond. Two types of glucans are elaborated.

1. Insoluble glucans (mutan) are polymers of predominantly α-1-3 linked glucose moieties split off from the sucrose. Mutant strains of *Strept. mutans* lacking the ability to synthesize insoluble α-1-3 linked glucan are comparatively less cariogenic.

2. Soluble glucans built up mainly of α-1-6 linked glucose which probably interlink the bacteria in plaque. Glucans comprise up to 10 per cent of the dry weight of plaque and present a barrier to external diffusion of acid produced by plaque bacteria from the glycolytic conversion of glucose to lactic acid. This glucose is largely derived from the hydrolysis of dietary sucrose by the bacterial enzyme invertase. The glucans also hinder the penetration of salivary buffers and presumably limit the antibacterial activity of antibodies, complement and PMNL.

3. Fructosyltransferase is an extracellular enzyme which also utilizes sucrose, but this time polymerizing the fructose subunits to produce fructans. Fructans do not persist long in plaque and may be a source of energy rather than a mechanism for adhesion to teeth.

4. Glycosidic hydrolases. Oral streptococci possess glycosidic hydrolases which cleave carbohydrates from salivary glycoproteins. The liberated sugars form an important energy source for the plaque bacteria between meals.

5. Dextranases enable the organism to metabolize the soluble glucans between meals. Mutant organisms lacking the dextranase glucano-hydrolase are not cariogenic.

The immunological aspects of dental caries

Anatomical factors do not favour the local defences against cariogenic bacteria. The susceptible enamel is acellular and has no blood supply. Opsonizing antibodies and PMNL can only gain access to the bacteria on the tooth surface via the crevicular fluid and saliva. The plaque itself forms a further barrier to successful elimination of the streptococci.

It was remarkable, therefore that patients with active caries were shown to have an altered antibody response to cariogenic bacteria, and the first reports that animals could be protected against caries by immunization alone were received with scepticism.

Innate immunity to caries

Can differences in the immune responsiveness of the individual to cariogenic bacteria account for the variations in susceptibility to caries which exist between subjects living on similar diets? No clear answer has yet emerged.

Although Challacombe (1980) and Kennedy and co-workers (1965) have reported that caries-free subjects had a raised serum (but not salivary) antibody titre to cell wall antigens of cariogenic streptococci, in another study young Dutch military recruits with untreated caries had high serum levels of antibody to *Strept. mutans* compared with those in colleagues who were caries free. The antibody titres were highest in the soldiers with high caries scores. Caries-free subjects had low levels of *Strept. mutans* in their dental plaque.

This disagreement regarding the protective value of naturally developing humoral immunity to cariogenic organisms may arise because researchers have tried to relate antibody titres to the number of decayed missing and filled teeth (DMF-T) in adults. The DMF index in adults is really a cumulative total of past experience of caries rather than a measure of current caries activity. The number of fresh lesions developing *per annum* (caries increment) in children soon after the eruption of the dentition is more relevant to the question of whether the immune response does naturally afford significant protection against caries.

Caries in immunodeficiency states

Knowledge of the caries susceptibility of patients with various types of immunodeficiency disorders would have some bearing on the question of whether the immune system can significantly control caries in humans and indicate the relative importance of the different components of the immune response.

The literature is not unanimous but the rare patients with profound immunodeficiencies ranging from agammaglobulinaemia to disorders of polymorphonuclear leucocytes seem to be somewhat more prone to caries than normal subjects (Fig. 2.3). Some patients with a selective deficiency of secretory IgA may be protected from caries by a compensatory production of secretory IgM in their saliva.

What is clear is that *Strept mutans* is only weakly immunogenic when it naturally accumulates as dental plaque in man or monkey. *Strept. mutans* is virtually confined to the surfaces of teeth and is seldom isolated and in only small numbers from the oral cavity before the teeth erupt. As a consequence, production of specific antibodies occurs too late and their blood level remains too low to protect teeth adequately against decay, particularly in their caries-susceptible phase just after eruption.

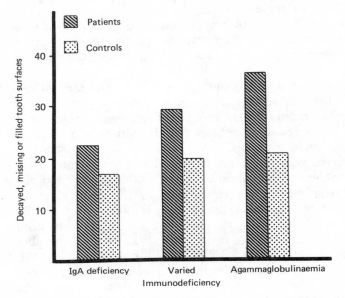

Fig. 2.3   Dental caries in immunodeficient patients. (From Legler, D. W., McGhee, J. R., Mestecky, J., Arnold, R. R. and Carson, J. Legler, D. W., (1980). *Journal of Dental Research* **59**, Special Issue B.)

In summary, the immune system does not seem to play a significant part in the control of tooth decay in the unimmunized human. The amount of sucrose in the diet, the frequency with which it is eaten and the concentration of fluoride in the drinking water seem to be of overriding importance.

Immunization against dental caries
Although Clarke identified *Streptococcus mutans* as the organism responsible for dental decay in 1924 this finding was not at first generally accepted, and the first attempts at protection of caries by immunization in 1934 employed a *Lactobacillus acidophilus* vaccine and were unsuccessful.

Subsequent experiments by Bowen in 1969 showing that monkeys could be protected against caries with vaccines prepared from *Strept. mutans* were particularly relevant to caries in humans. The teeth of these animals are similar in their morphology and sequences of eruption to those of man. Fissure and smooth surface lesions resembling those in human caries are induced when macaque monkeys with a normal mixed oral flora are given a human-type diet containing sucrose. On this diet, *Strept. mutans* colonizes the teeth, whereas this organism is usually absent from monkeys living in the wild state.

The similarities between the immune system of these monkeys and that of man make these animals particularly valuable models for evaluating vaccines intended for use in humans.

Routes for immunization

Subcutaneous or *submucosal* are the parenteral routes for inoculation of *Strept. mutans* which have afforded the best immunity against caries in monkeys and the protection correlated with the levels of specific serum IgG antibody, rather than of the titre of secretory IgA antibody in the saliva.

Oral mucosa   The topical application of immunizing concentrations of organisms to mucosal surfaces results in production of specific secretory IgA (s-IgA) rather than serum antibody.

Oral immunization by the addition of *Strept. mutans* to the drinking water significantly inhibited the induction of caries in rats but not in monkeys. This protection was associated with a rise in salivary secretory IgA streptococcal antibody.

Repeated application of the organisms to the gingivae of monkeys has proved a feeble method of immunostimulation and no protection ensued.

Salivary gland   The concept of preferentially stimulating a locally protective s-IgA response has been pursued by either injection of the vaccine into or near the major salivary glands or by instillation into their ducts. Levels of specific s-IgA can be produced in this way, sufficient to inhibit caries in rats but not monkeys.

Gastrointestinal tract   *Strept. mutans* has been implanted in the stomachs of monkeys and swallowed in capsules by human volunteers. Antistreptococcal s-IgA antibody production was stimulated in the saliva and streptococcal counts reduced in plaque.

As mentioned previously (Chapter 1), if the gut-associated lymphoid tissue (GALT) is stimulated with an immunogenic dose of swallowed bacteria, specific s-IgA production is induced in saliva and milk, i.e. in secretions produced remote from the original site of antigenic stimulation by precursor IgA-forming lymphoid cells 'homing' from the GALT to the salivary glands and breast.

The potential hazards of streptococcal vaccines

Upper respiratory tract infections by β-haemolytic Group A streptococci are occasionally followed by acute rheumatic fever or, alternatively, acute glomerulonephritis. These complications generally arise one to four weeks after the initial pharyngitis and coincide with a significant rise in the titre of streptococcal antibody in the patient's serum. Patients with rheumatic fever make antistreptococcal antibodies which cross-react with and are damaging to normal cardiac muscle. In post-streptococcal glomerulonephritis, the damage is mediated by the deposition of immune complexes in the kidney consisting of streptococcal antigens and antistreptococcal antibodies.

These observations suggest that in some patients the immune response to certain streptococci may be damaging as well as protective. Streptococci have a diversity of antigens, some of which confer protection and others which are responsible for the harmful sequelae. A *Strept. mutans* vaccine against caries should ideally be optimally protective in its antigenic composition whilst lacking non-protective or noxious antigens. Some of the antigens of *Strept. mutans* have now been defined and include the following.

Cell wall-associated polysaccharides
Bratthall (1969) classified strains of *Strept. mutans* serologically on the basis of cell wall polysaccharide antigens. Eight *Strept. mutans* serotypes (*a* to *h*) have been described and the *c* and *d* strains are the most important strains associated with human caries.

Cell wall-associated protein antigens
Since vaccines made from the cell wall alone protect monkeys against caries, the major protective antigens may well be located in this part of the coccus. Although two cell wall-associated protein antigens, named A and B have been described other antigens remain to be purified, and exactly which of the cell wall antigen(s) may be important for protection is not yet known.

Protein I/II
This purified protein with two sets of antigenic determinants I and II present in the supernatant of cultures of *Strept. mutans* has been shown by Lehner, Russell and Caldwell (1980) to be an effective vaccine against tooth decay in monkeys.

Enzymes
These include glucosyltransferases and fructosyltransferases. Experiments attempting to prevent caries in monkeys by immunization with enzyme preparations have only been occasionally successful. Immunization with glycosidic hydrolases has effected some reduction in the caries rate.

Glucan receptor protein

This protein acts as a ligand or binding site on the streptococcus for the glucans it produces, and serves to aggregate the organisms proliferating on tooth surfaces. Immunization with this protein might furnish antibodies capable of blocking the binding site and preventing colonization of the enamel.

Undesirable streptococcal antigens

Van de Rijn *et al.* (1976) showed that an antiserum raised in rabbits against *Strept. mutans* contained antibodies which could also bind to normal human myocardium. One of these streptococcal antigens cross-reacting with heart muscle is the cell wall-associated antigen B.

However, not all antimyocardial antibodies lead to tissue damage. Further, *Strept. mutans* is not a cause of acute rheumatic fever or glomerulonephritis in man; nor have these diseases developed in the non-human primates vaccinated with the organism.

Effector mechanisms in induced immunity to caries

How does the caries vaccine protect?

The ability to generate an adequate blood level of antistreptococcal antibody seems to be the most important requirement of an effective caries vaccine (Fig. 2.4). When monkeys were immunized parenterally with *Strept. mutans* by the intravenous, subcutaneous or intramuscular route, antibodies appeared in the blood, crevicular exudate and saliva.

The reduction in caries was correlated with the serum but not salivary antibody titre to *Strept. mutans*. In immunized monkeys, the reduction in caries was associated with a marked reduction in the density of *Strept. mutans* in the crevicular fluid and crevicular plaque. The streptococcal counts in the supragingival plaque and the saliva did not fall in the same striking manner. This suggested that approximal caries was inhibited as a result of a reduction in *Strept. mutans* at the necks of the teeth by antibodies arriving there in the crevicular exudate rather than in saliva.

Antibody probably mediates its effect by opsonizing the bacteria making them more readily phagocytosable by the PMNLs emanating from the gingival crevice. These leucocytes are equipped with a receptor for the Fc tails of IgG antibodies bound to the bacteria. Further, complement activation by the IgG–bacterium complex can lead to deposition of the C3 complement component on the cell surface leading to opsonization via the C3 receptor of PMNL (Fig. 2.5).

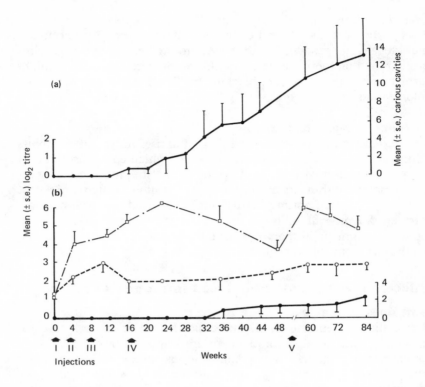

Fig. 2.4 Specific antibody response and protection against caries in monkeys immunized against *Streptococcus mutans*. Sequential serum and salivary antibody responses to immunization in rhesus monkeys: **(a)** sham-immunized (saline) **(b)** immunized. (Reprinted by kind permission from Lehner, T. *et al. Nature*, **254**, 517–20. Copyright 1975, Macmillan Journals Limited.)

When rhesus monkeys were given intravenous infusions of immune plasma containing antibodies against *Strept. mutans* of the three major immunoglobulin classes IgG, IgM and IgA, no protection from caries resulted. However, passive transfer of only the IgG fraction of this immune serum significantly prevented caries in these animals. The explanation put forward was that in the unfractionated serum which failed to provide passive immunity, the IgA component could have interfered with the usual opsonizing activity of the IgG antibody, possibly by competing for sites on the bacteria.

Secretory IgA protects in a different way. It combines with oral micro-organisms and effectively prevents their adherence to either enamel or oral epithelium (Fig. 2.5). These antigen–antibody complexes are then swept away by the salivary flow during eating and are swallowed. This process of antigen disposal by secretory IgA forms an attractive basis for immunization against caries. In theory, the selective stimulation of a predominantly secretory type of immunity by a topical *Strept. mutans* vaccine need not involve the production of IgG serum antibody with the attendant risks of acute glomerulonephritis and rheumatic fever. However, to date only rats have been effectively immunized against caries by this approach.

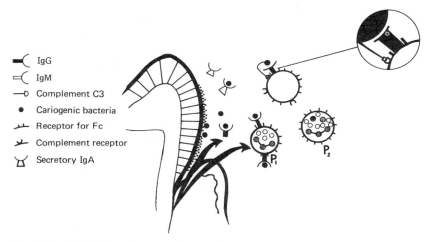

Fig. 2.5 Mechanisms for protections against cariogenic bacteria. IgG and IgM antibody and complement C3 in the crevicular exudate opsonize cariogenic bacteria which are then more efficiently phagocytosed by crevicular polymorphonuclear leucocytes (P_1) and subsequently killed intracellularly (P_2). The polymorph has a specific receptor for the Fc end of the IgG molecule and also a complement receptor. Secretory IgA in the saliva combines with bacteria and inhibits their adherence to the tooth surface. (Diagram not to scale.)

More than 90 per cent of the inflammatory cells in the crevicular fluid are PMNL. There is a continuous traffic of blood PMNLs from the gingival capillaries into the gingival crevice where they form the main phagocytes in the crevicular exudate. Small numbers of phagocytic monocytes complete this task force. About one-quarter of the crevicular PMNL are effete but the remainder are viable and functional and often contain ingested bacteria. They are as capable as blood PMNL of phagocytosing and killing *Strept. mutans*. Only half of the leucocytes in saliva are viable and their powers of phagocytosis are less than crevicular and blood PMNLs.

In monkeys immunized with *Strept. mutans*, the opsonizing activity of crevicular fluid samples and serum, enhancing PMNL phagocytosis of *Strept. mutans*, was significantly greater than that from non-immune animals. Saliva had less opsonizing activity.

Future prospects for a caries vaccine

At present, the prevention of caries in man by immunization is only an attractive proposition. Before clinical trials in humans can commence, we need to produce a purified highly immunogenic preparation of an exclusively protective antigen, if such exists. Some of the regimes for successful protection of monkeys have employed intravenous injections or have needed to use Freund's incomplete adjuvant to boost antibody levels. Neither of these manoeuvres is suitable for use in humans. Effective induction of secretory immunity by topical application or ingestion of the immunogen as a means of vaccination is further from fruition.

Although it occasions pain and time lost from work for many, dental caries is not a serious or life-threatening disorder. When the present low acceptance rates by the general public for vaccines against potentially lethal infections are considered, it is obvious that more research is necessary before an entirely safe and effective caries vaccine acceptable for general use becomes a practical reality.

Pulpal and periapical conditions

Pulpitis

At an early stage in dental caries, possibly when the lesion is still confined to the enamel, an inflammatory reaction takes place in the underlying pulp; before organisms have reached the pulp. Carious dentine sealed in cavities prepared in sound teeth excites the same inflammatory response. It seems then that bacterial products diffusing through enamel and dentine are responsible for this early localized pulpitis.

There is experimental evidence that the intensity of the pulpal response depends upon the immune status of the host. When monkeys previously sensitized to bovine serum albumin by a systemic route had this antigen subsequently applied to the floors of deep cavities prepared in their teeth, an acute pulpitis, occasionally even a total pulpal necrosis, resulted. The monkey teeth showed little reaction to the cavity procedure alone. Unimmunized animals showed only a minimal pulpal reaction to application of the antigen.

We do not yet have formal proof that, in humans, the immune

reaction to the cariogenic bacteria will influence the extent or severity of the pulpal reaction to dental caries. Cases of immunodeficient patients with microbial invasion of the pulp due to caries are on record in which the usual cellular infiltrate was noticeably absent. The pulp undergoes the same inflammatory changes as any other connective tissue in the body in response to endotoxins and other bacterial products, but drainage of the exudate and normal recovery of the pulp is undoubtedly hindered by the peculiar situation of the pulp confined within a rigid pulp chamber.

In an early pulpitis the inflammatory features are restricted to a small area of the coronal pulp (an acute partial pulpitis). Lymphocytes and monocytes are the predominant cell types in the sparse infiltrate (Fig. 2.6). Later, PMNL accumulate in significant numbers and a small coronal abscess may result.

The pathogenesis of pulpitis may be explained by local activation of complement, either directly by endotoxin or by complexes of antibody and bacterial antigens. Binding of the C3b activation product to the receptors of macrophages and PMNL stimulates the macrophages to release the proteolytic enzyme collagenase and the polymorphonuclear leucocytes their lysosomal enzymes, resulting in local destruction of pulpal tissue. Endotoxin can also directly stimulate macrophages to produce collagenase.

As the carious cavity enlarges, further destruction of the dentine takes place and eventually the pulp is invaded by cariogenic bacteria. Large numbers of macrophages, lymphocytes and plasma cells, characteristic of a chronic inflammatory cell population, infiltrate the necrotic pulp tissue. This infiltrate contains cells forming antibody, mostly of the IgG class. The specificity of this locally synthesized antibody remains to be determined, but presumably it is directed against the cariogenic bacteria.

Periapical granuloma

A periapical granuloma consists of granulation tissue forming around the apex of a non-vital tooth and is a chronic inflammatory response to endotoxins from bacteria sequestered in the pulpless root canal largely out of reach of PMNL and macrophages. The periapical granuloma is intensely infiltrated by lymphocytes and plasma cells, together with macrophages and PMNL which phagocytose bacteria emerging from the apical foramen of the tooth. As a consequence, periapical granulomas are generally sterile. Plasma cells producing IgG and lesser numbers of the IgA- and IgM-producing cells have been demonstrated in this granuloma by direct immunofluorescence.

34

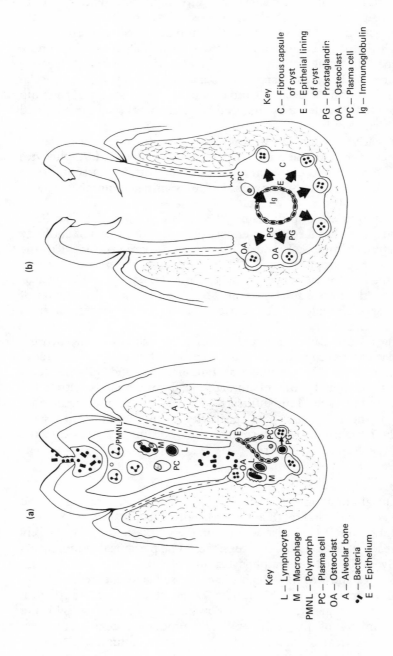

Fig. 2.6 Cell-mediated immunity in pulpal and periapical disease. **(a)** Periapical granuloma. **(b)** Dental cyst.

Key

L — Lymphocyte
M — Macrophage
PMNL — Polymorph
PC — Plasma cell
OA — Osteoclast
A — Alveolar bone
•, — Bacteria
E — Epithelium

Key

C — Fibrous capsule
 of cyst
E — Epithelial lining
 of cyst
PG — Prostaglandin:
OA — Osteoclast
PC — Plasma cell
Ig — Immunobulin

Although in skilled hands the obliteration of the pulp canals of dead teeth by a root filling is remarkably successful failures of endodontic treatment do occur. A better understanding of the nature of the pathological processes occurring in the periapical granuloma might suggest pharmacological methods or antibacterial agents for improving the success of root canal therapy. The specificity of the infiltrate and the bacteria responsible for the reaction have not been established. It is also not known whether the immune reaction is due to immune complex formation or to cell-mediated immunity.

Dental cyst

The epithelial rests of Malassez included in the periapical granuloma may proliferate and in time degenerate to form a dental cyst (apical periodontal cyst). The young cyst is lined by a hyperplastic stratified squamous epithelium supported by a capsule of collagen fibres. The fibrous capsule is infiltrated by a mixed population of lymphocytes plasma cells macrophages and PMNL (Fig. 2.6). Toller and Holborow (1969) identified three major classes of immunoglobulin—IgA, IgG, IgM—in the cyst fluid. The concentrations of IgA and IgG were significantly higher in the cyst fluid than in serum. These antibodies are probably produced locally by the plasma cells in the cyst capsule (Fig. 2.6), although some may be derived from the blood. The immunoglobulin classes of the plasma cells corresponded with the respective levels of these proteins in the cyst fluid.

Prostaglandins in jaw cysts

Prostaglandins were discovered in the walls of dental and dentigerous (follicular) cysts by Harris *et al.* (1973). The prostaglandin is thought to be elaborated in the fibrous capsule of the cyst rather than in its epithelial lining. Prostaglandins synthesized by the cyst were shown to be capable of activating osteoclasts in an animal system to resorb bone (Fig. 2.6). This represents one mechanism by which cysts expand within the jaws. Bacterial antigens and mitogens can also stimulate lymphocytes to secrete a soluble lymphokine, osteoclast-activating factor which then can mediate osteoclastic resorption of bone. Finally, bacterial endotoxins are also capable of inhibiting bone growth *in vitro* which would achieve the same result.

Immunological reactions to dental materials

The cell-mediated reaction to eugenol is one of the few convincing examples of adverse immunological reactions to dental materials in common use.

An inflammatory reaction of the mucosa in contact with an eugenol-containing pack applied after periodontal surgery occurs with increasing frequency and severity according to the number of occasions on which individual patients receive the periodontal dressing. It should be noted that eugenol is capable of acting both as a primary irritant (i.e. causes some slight non-immunological tissue reaction in all individuals) and as a secondary sensitizer in that a few patients will exhibit a marked cell-mediated contact stomatitis reaction (as above) presumably mediated by sensitized lymphocytes.

Cinnamon acetonide, a flavouring ingredient, has been responsible for a contact stomatitis reaction to a toothpaste, again only occurring in a small minority of users, and confirmed by patch testing to be a delayed hypersensitivity reaction (cell mediated).

In cell-mediated reactions, the reaction is most pronounced one to two days after contact with the antigen, hence the term delayed-type hypersensitivity. Usually, these reactions are provoked by the antigen binding to the host's cells and altering their surface structure—the cell-mediated response is directed at these modified autologous cells.

In the patch test, the suspected agent, incorporated in an inert base such as paraffin, is applied to the skin. In a positive test, a vesicular inflammatory reaction appears in the skin in contact with the agent, within forty-eight hours (Fig. 2.7).

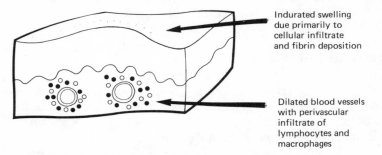

Indurated swelling
due primarily to
cellular infiltrate
and fibrin deposition

Dilated blood vessels
with perivascular
infiltrate of
lymphocytes and
macrophages

Fig. 2.7   The delayed hypersensitivity reaction is the basis of two diagnostic tests.
(a) The patch test. The topical application of a substance, e.g. dinitrochlorobenzene (DNCB), in a person sensitized to the material by a previous application.
(b) The tuberculin test. Intradermal injection of purified protein derivative (PPD)
from *Mycobacterium tuberculosis* in a person. A positive reaction occurs in
(i) patients with tuberculosis, (ii) patients who have recovered from tuberculosis,
(iii) subjects immunized with Bacille Calmette-Guérin vaccine (BCG).

Allergic reactions to denture base materials such as methyl methacrylate are extremely rare and the common denture stomatitis is usually due to candidal colonization of the fitting surface. Even dental technicians constantly handling the mixture of resin monomer are more liable to a primary irritant 'wear and tear' type of dermatitis confined to the hands, than any allergic reaction. Similarly, alloys containing chromium, nickel and cobalt are apparently inert as denture base materials, whereas these metals are amongst the commonest agents to be incriminated in contact dermatitis associated with jewellery or buckles or as ingredients in building cement.

Materials implanted beneath the mucosa in direct contact with the connective tissue, such as in root fillings and metal implants or bone plates, might, on the face of it, be more immunogenic in these sites, but evidence linking failure of root treatment or implants with immunological reactions to the dental materials involved is entirely lacking.

References

Bowen, W. H. (1969). A vaccine against dental caries. A pilot experiment in monkeys (Macaca Irus). *British Dental Journal* **126**, 159–60.

Bratthall, D. (1969). Demonstration of five serological groups of streptococcal strains resembling *Streptococcus mutans*. *Odontologisk Revy* **21**, 143–52.

Challacombe, S. J. (1980). Serum and salivary antibodies to *Streptococcus mutans* in relation to the development and treatment of human dental caries. *Archives of Oral Biology* **25**, 495–502.

Clarke, J. K. (1924). Bacterial factor in the aetiology of dental caries. *British Journal of Experimental Pathology* **5**, 141–7.

Harris, M., Jenkins, M. V., Bennett, A. and Wills, M. R. (1973). Prostaglandin production and bone resorption by dental cysts. *Nature* **245**, 213–15.

Kennedy, A. E., Shklar, J. A., Hayashi, J. A. and Bahn, A. N. (1965). Antibodies to cariogenic streptococci in humans. *Archives of Oral Biology* **13**, 1275–8.

Lehner, T., Russell, M. W. and Caldwell, J. (1980). Immunisation with a purified protein from *Streptococcus mutans* against dental caries in rhesus monkeys. *Lancet* **i**, 995–6.

Toller, P. A. and Holborow, E. J. (1969). Immunoglobulins and immunoglobulin-containing cells in cysts of the jaws. *Lancet* **ii**, 178–81.

Van de Rijn, I., Bleiweis, A. S. and Zabriskie, J. B. (1976). Antigens in *Streptococcus mutans* cross reactive with human heart muscle. *Journal of Dental Research* **55**, C59–64.

Further reading

Dental caries

Arnold, R. R., Prince, S. J., Mestecky, J., Lynch, D., Lynch, M. and McGhee, J. R. (1978). Secretory immunity and immunodeficiency. In

Secretory immunity and infection, pp. 401–410 Advances in Experimental Medicine and Biology. Vol. 107, Ed. by J. R. McGhee, J. Mestecky and J. L. Babb, Plenum Press, New York and London.

Cohen, B., Colman, G. and Russell, R. R. B. (1979). Immunisation against dental caries. Further studies. *British Dental Journal* **147**, 9–14.

Gibbons, R. J. (1980). Adhesion of bacteria to the surfaces of the mouth. In *Microbial adhesion to surfaces*, Proceedings of a symposium, Reading University, pp. 1–21. Ed. by R. C. W. Berkeley, J. M. Lynch, J. Melling, P. R. Rutter and B. Vincent. Ellis Morwood, Chichester.

Huis, 'In't Veld, J., Bannet, D. van Palenstein, Helderman, W., Sampaio Camargo, P. and Backer-Dirks, O. (1978). Antibodies against *Streptococcus mutans* and glucosyltransferases in caries-free and caries-active military recruits. in *Secretory Immunity and Infection*, pp. 369–81. Advances in Experimental Medicine and Biology, Vol. 107. Ed. by J. R. McGhee, J. Mestecky and J. L. Babb. Plenum Press, New York and London.

Lehner, R., Challacombe, S. J., Wilton, J. M. A. and Caldwell, J. (1976). Cellular and humoral immune responses in vaccination against dental caries in monkeys. *Nature* **264**, 69–72.

Michalek, S. M., McGhee, J. R., Mestecky, J., Arnold, R. R. and Bozzo, L. (1976). Ingestion of *Streptococcus mutans* induces secretory immunoglobulin A and caries immunity. *Science* **192**, 1238–40.

Scully, C. M. and Lehner, T. (1979). Opsonisation, phagocytosis and killing of *Streptococcus mutans* by polymorphonuclear leukocytes in relation to dental caries in the rhesus monkey (macaca mulatta). *Archives of Oral Biology* **24**, 307–312.

Pulpal and periapical conditions

Bergenholtz, G., Ahlstedt, S. and Lindhe, J. (1977). Experimental pulpitis in immunized monkeys. *Scandinavian Journal of Dental Research* **85**, 396–406.

Horton, J. E., Raisz, L. G., Simmons, H. A., Oppenheim, J. J. and Mergenhagen, S. E. (1972). Bone resorbing activity in supernatant fluid from human cultured peripheral blood leukocytes. *Science* **177**, 793–5.

Morse, D. R. (1977). Immunologic aspects of pulpal-periapical diseases. A review. *Oral Surgery* **43**, 436–51.

Pulver, W. H., Taubman, M. A. and Smith, D. J. (1977). Immune components in normal and inflamed human dental pulp. *Archives of Oral Biology* **22**, 103–111.

Torneck, C. D. (1974). Changes in the fine structure of the pulp in human caries pulpitis. 2. Inflammatory infiltrate. *Journal of Oral Pathology* **3**, 83–99.

Cysts

Toller, P. A. (1971). Immunological factors in cysts of the jaw. *Journal of the Royal Society of Medicine* **64**, 556–9.

Immune reaction to dental materials

Koch, G., Magnusson, B. and Nyquist, G. (1971). Contact allergy to medicaments and materials used in dentistry. *Odontologisk Revy* **22**, 275–89.

3

Periodontal Disease

There is considerable evidence that the accumulation of bacterial plaque at the necks of the teeth causes gingivitis. Early plaque is predominantly coccal and Gram-positive, containing such organisms as *Strept. mutans* and *Strept. sanguis*. Plaque which has been allowed to accumulate is predominantly Gram-negative and contains a greater proportion of filamentous, rod-shaped and spirochaetal organisms. In view of the large variety of bacteria present, it seems unlikely that the disease is due to a specific organism. Although mono-infection of experimental animals can produce gingivitis and periodontal disease, extrapolation of these results to the human situation is difficult. Indeed, periodontal disease has been observed in germ-free animals. The immune response to specific bacteria found in dental plaque has been examined in patients with periodontal disease on the assumption that bacteria which produce an enhanced immune response during the course of the disease are causally associated with the disease.

The damaging effects of dental bacterial plaque upon the periodontium

Direct effects of plaque
Since gingivitis in the human occurs when bacterial plaque accumulates there is a strong inference that the bacteria are *directly* responsible for the disease.

In vitro experiments have shown that extracts of dental bacterial plaque are harmful to tissue culture cells and it can be inferred that the barrier role of the gingival epithelium is reduced by this effect. A large number of enzymes are produced by the bacteria (hyaluronidase, elastase, collagenase and probably cathepsin D) and these may increase the permeability of the epithelium allowing other toxic products of the bacteria to penetrate to the underlying tissue.

The predominantly Gram-negative flora which occurs with the onset of gingivitis contains a higher proportion of endotoxin than that of the normally occurring Gram-positive flora. A positive correlation between the level of endotoxin in the dental plaque and the degree of gingivitis has been shown, so that this material may be important in the onset and progression of the disease. Endotoxin has a range of harmful effects some mediated by immunological mechanisms. It may:

(i) cause direct cell injury with inhibition of protein synthesis, disruption of mitochondria and release of lysosomal enzymes;

(ii) activate the complement and kinin systems;

(iii) cause vasoconstriction via release of catecholamines;

(iv) cause intravascular coagulation;

(v) promote separation of the epithelial cells, thus increasing epithelial permeability; a reduction in adhesiveness of epithelial cells has been shown *in vitro*.

Indirect effects of plaque
In addition to the direct effect of dental plaque, the material has also been shown to contain materials with effects on the gingiva which act through or on immune mechanisms.

Mitogenic effect
A mitogen is a substance which induces mitosis. In relation to the lymphocyte, mitogens trigger mitosis and differentiation just like specific antigen. Apparently, this phenomenon is dependent upon the interaction of the mitogen with surface receptors on the lymphocyte, but in a non-specific manner, the interaction being entirely unrelated to the antigenic specificity of the lymphocyte. Phytohaemagglutinin, concanavalin A and pokeweed mitogen are mitogens of plant origin that are frequently used in lymphocyte culture to demonstrate the responsive state of the lymphocytes.

The principal mitogens of dental plaque are levan, dextran and endotoxin. The direct effect of these mitogens appears to be on B lymphocytes, not T lymphocytes. In fact, they are also called *polyclonal B cell stimulators or activators*. This anomalous situation, in which a B lymphocyte is stimulated other than by its particular antigen, may lead to antibody production. It can be seen that such a response of the gingiva would lead to proliferation of antibody-forming cells directed against a range of bacterial and other antigens not specifically associated with dental plaque.

B cell mitogens also induce the production of lymphokines by B cells. The study of this phenomenon has been facilitated by the fact that T and B lymphocytes may be separated by several methods (Fig. 3.1).

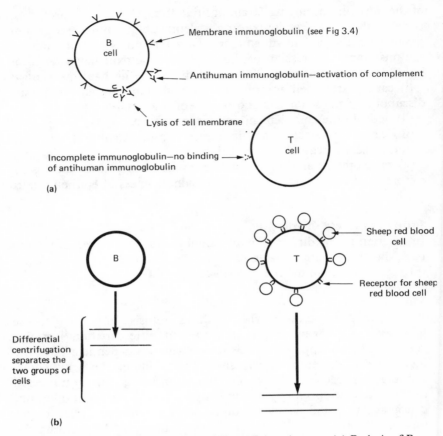

Fig. 3.1   Methods for the separation of T and B lymphocytes. **(a)** By lysis of B cells with antihuman immunoglobulin serum in the presence of complement. **(b)** By rosette formation. The lymphocytes are incubated with sheep red blood cells.

(a) Incubation of lymphocytes with certain anti-immunoglobulin sera followed by complement leads to the lysis of cells bearing large amounts of immunoglobulin on the surface, i.e. B lymphocytes, leaving the T lymphocytes intact.

(b) The T lymphocytes have receptors for sheep red cells on their surface, with which they form rosettes; this is an empirical observation and its physiological significance is obscure. Thus incubation of the T and B lymphocytes with sheep red blood cells, followed by differential centrifugation leads to the separation of the two populations of lymphocytes, since the T cells with attached erythrocytes are denser.

One important lymphokine synthesized by T and B lymphocytes is osteoclast-activating factor, which has been shown to be capable of stimulating osteoclasts in culture to resorb bone by a mechanism apparently independent of prostaglandin synthesis. Thus, by a roundabout route, the polyclonal B cell activators of dental plaque may stimulate osteoclasts adjacent to the alveolar bone to resorb the supporting bone of the tooth.

In addition to effects on B cells, B cell mitogens also apparently influence the T cell response to dental plaque antigen, either suppressing or amplifying the response depending upon the manner or order of presentation of the mitogen and the antigen. This phenomenon may explain the immunopotentiating effect of dental plaque observed in experimental gingivitis described below.

It has been noticed in several investigations in which plaque was allowed to accumulate that the response of peripheral blood lymphocytes to the mitogen phytohaemagglutinin and to antigens unrelated to dental plaque was enhanced with the accumulation of dental plaque and the resultant onset of gingivitis. The reason for this immunopotentiating effect of dental plaque is not clear, but the phenomenon may lead to immune responses to additional unrelated antigens in the periodontium.

Immunological evidence incriminating certain micro-organisms in periodontal disease

Antibody response

It was at one time argued that an elevation in the level of antibody directed against a particular organism occurring during the course of a disease was evidence that the organism was causally associated with the disease. This is not always true and in periodontal disease there are a number of other difficulties which must be taken into account.

1. There is a large variety of bacteria and their antigens present in the plaque, except for in the case of acute ulcerative gingivitis when two bacterial strains predominate. However, certain bacteria increase disproportionately in periodontal disease and more attention has been paid to the antibody level relating to these organisms.

2. Some bacteria have proved extremely difficult to isolate in pure culture.

3. Measurements of the concentrations of the serum antibody to bacteria in patients may not represent the situation in the gingival lesion itself.

Antibody levels in the serum have been measured using agglutination of antigen-coated red cells, immunodiffusion through agar and a quantitative adaptation of the fluorescent antibody technique. The levels in saliva have also been measured. A list of the

Table 3.1   Bacterial species examined in studies of the immune response to organisms of dental plaque. Where an enhanced response has been detected, for example with the organisms marked* under lymphoblastic response, it may be thought to implicate that organism in the pathogenesis of the disease. As is explained in the text, this is not always the case. Note how many organisms give an enhanced lymphoblastic response.

Serum antibody levels	Lymphoblastic response
Leptotrichia buccalis	*Bacteroides melaninogenicus* *
Bacteroides melaninogenicus	*Actinomyces israelii* *
Actinomyces israelii	*Actinomyces naeslundii* *
Actinomyces naeslundii	*Veillonella alcalescens* *
Bacterionema matruchotii	*Actinomyces viscosus* *
Eubacterium saburreum	*Arachnia propionica* *
Fusibacterium nucleatum	*Streptococcus sanguis*
Treponema macrodentium	*Fusibacterium nucleatum*
	Lactobacillus acidophilus
	Proteus mirabilis

organisms examined is given in Table 3.1 and although not exhaustive, this gives some indication of the task. In general, antibody titres are raised in subjects with chronic periodontal disease but the individual variation within the subjects suffering from the disease does not allow for the drawing of a correlation between the disease and the raised antibody titre. Thus, antibody titres as high as those found in patients with periodontal disease occur also in normal subjects and this response is probably due to bacteria bearing similar antigens being found elsewhere in the body, presumably in the gut. Despite this assumption of cross-reactivity between gut organisms and those organisms found in relation to periodontal disease, remarkably little information is available which does demonstrate such cross-reactivity.

Cell-mediated responses
The antigens of dental plaque bacteria may also evoke a cellular immune response. In most studies, one of the following three *in vitro* methods has been employed.

1. The inhibition of leucocyte or macrophage migration.
2. The measurement of the cytotoxic effect of stimulated lymphocytes.
3. The assessment of lymphocyte transformation.

The interaction of T lymphocyte with antigen leads to the production of a range of lymphokines amongst which is MIF, the lymphokine which reduces macrophage migration (Fig. 3.2). Peritoneal exudate macrophages from a laboratory animal may

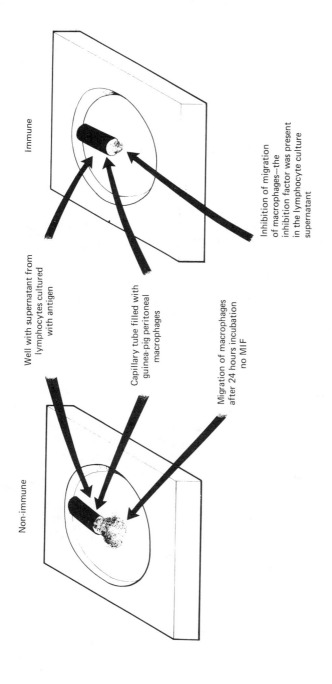

Non-immune

Immune

Well with supernatant from
lymphocytes cultured
with antigen

Capillary tube filled with
guinea-pig peritoneal
macrophages

Migration of macrophages
after 24 hours incubation
no MIF

Inhibition of migration
of macrophages—the
inhibition factor was present
in the lymphocyte culture
supernatant

Fig. 3.2 Migration inhibition factor (MIF).

be used as the indicator cell or, alternatively, the granulocytes of the buffy coat of the blood of the individual being examined (leucocyte migration inhibition, LMI). In the first case, the supernatant from antigen-stimulated lymphocyte cultures is transferred to wells containing peritoneal exudate macrophages in capillary tubes. Normally, the macrophages migrate out of the capillary during overnight incubation. The area of migration of the macrophages from the tubes is compared with that observed when supernatants from unstimulated cultures have been employed. With LMI, the responding lymphocytes and indicator cells, the granulocytes, are together in the same tube.

Using these assays, production of MIF has been shown to occur *in vitro* in lymphocytes taken from patients with periodontal disease in response to antigens of plaque bacteria. It has also been shown to be reduced below normal in idiopathic juvenile periodontitis in children and adolescents, despite the fact that the other parameters of the cellular immune response appear normal. This lack of production of MIF has been interpreted as a contributory factor to this unusual form of periodontal disease.

Interaction of antigen with T lymphocytes may also lead to the production of a soluble toxic material—lymphotoxin—which is non-specifically cytopathic or cytotoxic to many cell types; however, the lymphocytes themselves do not appear to be affected. Again, the production of lymphotoxin by lymphocytes stimulated by dental plaque antigen appears to correlate with the clinical severity of periodontal disease.

The *in vitro* correlate of cell-mediated immunity most widely examined in periodontal disease is that of lymphocyte transformation, that is, the characteristic change which takes place in the specifically sensitized T lymphocyte upon interaction with antigen. Changes may be assessed visually (Fig. 3.3) or more conveniently by the measurement of the uptake of radio-actively labelled nucleotides used in DNA synthesis. The lymphocyte response or stimulation index is a comparison of the uptake of this radiolabelled nucleotide with dental plaque antigen with that occurring with saline. Again, responses in periodontal disease are raised to both a variety of bacterial antigens of dental plaque (Table 3.1) and to extracts of dental plaque itself. In several studies in which the patient's own serum was included in the reaction mixture, the responses in severe disease were found to be comparable with the control subjects. This situation could be altered by substituting in the culture the sera of patients who had less severe periodontal disease. It was inferred that in severe disease the higher titre of antibody to antigens of dental plaque may be associated with immune complex formation, so that the antigen was no longer available for stimulation of the lymphocytes. The lymphocyte

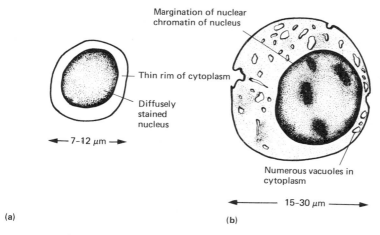

Fig. 3.3 (a) Circulating lymphocyte. (b) Lymphoblast.

response to the dental plaque antigens declines with an increase in age but the effect of removal of the teeth and treatment of periodontal disease has produced conflicting findings, so that the value of the test in implicating one or more organisms in the aetiology of the disease has not been substantiated.

The inflammatory infiltrate in periodontal disease

Much of the support for the assumption that the immune response to the dental plaque is of importance in the progression of periodontal disease has been derived from a study of the changes which occur in the inflammatory infiltrate during the course of the disease. Clinically normal gingiva possesses a small population of lymphocytes, plasma cells and macrophages which becomes evident at the time of the eruption of the tooth. The lymphoid population of the gingiva changes with the induction of gingivitis and periodontal disease. The evidence that such changes occur has been derived from light and electron microscopy as well as the fluorescent antibody technique.

In the early stages of inflammation the infiltrate is predominantly small mononuclear cells with fewer PMNLs, mast cells and macrophages. The majority of the lymphocytes appear to be T cells. With increasing severity of disease, the infiltrate has an increasing proportion of B lymphocytes and plasma cells. In established periodontal disease the majority of the plasma cells are producing IgG. There are four sub-classes of IgG1−4 —and not all of these four are represented in the gingival inflammatory infiltrate; IgG 2 is lacking or present in negligible amounts.

The fluorescent antibody technique (see Fig. 1.11) has also been used to assess the lymphocytes which bear immunoglobulin on the surface, that is, B cells. Immunoglobulin on the surface of the cell has to be distinguished from that which may be attached to the lymphocyte by an Fc receptor (Fig. 3.4). The latter immunoglobulin may be removed from the section by washing, whereas the immunoglobulin within the lymphocyte membrane remains during the washing process.

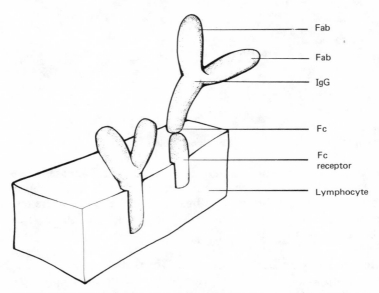

Fab

Fab

IgG

Fc

Fc receptor

Lymphocyte

Fig. 3.4   Two mechanisms by which IgG may be associated with the lymphocyte surface: the one on the left is intrinsic IgG produced by the lymphocyte; that on the right is merely attached to the Fc receptor in the lymphocyte membrane. The shape of the IgG molecule is more likely to be spherical. (From Mackler, B. F., Waldrop, T. C., Schur, P., Robertson, S. E. and Siraganian, R. P. (1978). *Journal of Periodontal Research* **13**, 109–19.)

In periodontitis the immunoglobulin class distribution of the plasma cell population is similar to that of the immunoglobulin-bearing lymphocytes which preceded it.

It might be presumed that plasma cells of the gingiva are producing immunoglobulin directed against the bacteria of the gingival crevice. However, it has been difficult to demonstrate a direct relationship between the immunoglobulins of the gingiva and the antigens of dental plaque bacteria. Such a situation is not uncommon at sites of chronic inflammation in response to bacterial infection. Thus, tonsillar inflammation evoked by one particular organism is accompanied by the proliferation of cells producing antibody against other bacteria. Again, the role of the polyclonal B cell activators described above must also be considered.

Macrophages are also present in significant numbers within the inflammatory infiltrate. They are detectable with histochemical techniques by their content of lysosomal hydrolases.

The role of the immune response in the aetiology of periodontal disease

In recent years, it has been proposed that at least part of the damage occurring in the periodontium is due to the immune response to the antigens of the dental bacterial plaque. This damage occurring from the immune response may occur in one of two ways. Firstly, the normal 'protective' mechanisms of the immune response may also lead to damage to the patient. The ways in which this may occur are as follows.

Reaginic reactions
The interaction of IgE, attached to the surface of a mast cell or basophil, with the appropriate antigen leads to the release of a range of pharmacologically active compounds—histamine, slow reactive substance A, prostaglandins, permeability and eosinophil chemotactic factors. This results in locally increased dilatation and permeability of blood vessels, allowing more ready access to the site by other types of antibody and phagocytic cells. If abnormally high amounts of IgE are formed against, for example, plaque antigens, an uncontrolled reaction could occur within the gingivae with oedema and tissue eosinophilia resulting. The total number of mast cells in inflamed gingiva appears to rise, but a more careful examination shows that in areas of increased inflammatory cell infiltrate the number of detectable mast cells is less. A reduction in the number of mast cells, based on an assessment using stains to detect mast cell granules, leads to the inference that these granules have been discharged, that is, that the cell has been activated by antigen. Experiments with isolated mast cells have led to the conclusion that the discharge of mast cell granules in periodontal disease is more likely to be the result of a direct effect of dental plaque rather than the classical combination of antigen of dental plaque with cytophilic IgE on the surface of the mast cell.

Complement activation
The complement system (Fig. 3.5) comprises a number of proteins, some of which have enzyme activity. Activation of the first component

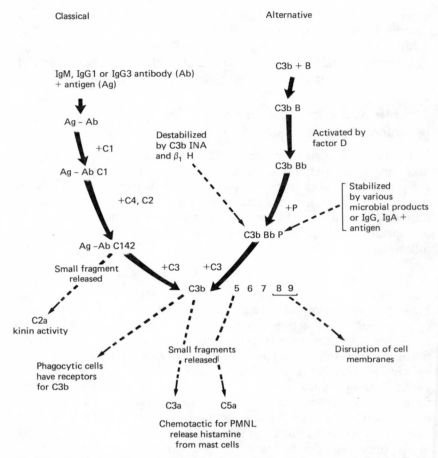

Fig 3.5 Activation of complement via the classical and alternative pathways. This is a cascade system with the components being assembled on the antigen surface (say, the bacterium) leading to death of the bacterium either by direct lysis by C8, C9 or by phagocytosis and intracellular killing of phagocytic cells. Notice C3 is being continuously slowly degraded with the production of C3b and, as a result, the alternative pathway is being continuously primed, although normally this is checked by C3b INA and β_1H. Substances which activate the alternative pathway do so by stabilizing C3b. Bb. P and so overriding the effects of C3b INA and β_1H.

in the sequence results in activation of several molecules of the next and so on, producing a 'landslide' effect. The classical pathway is most efficiently triggered by IgM antibodies, although IgG antibodies of the IgG 1 and IgG 3 subclasses are also effective. Antibodies of the IgA class and all four subclasses of IgG, as well as certain micro-organisms in the abscence of antibody, can trigger the alternative pathway.

As a result of this activation, the complement components are arranged on the antigen surface, although some of the enzyme liberated fragments, e.g. C3a and C5a anaphylatoxins, are liberated into free solution, leading to a local increase in capillary permeability and an attraction of PMNL to the site of complement activation. The C8 component on the antigen surface, with the help of C9, may damage a cell membrane on which the antigen resides. Were this to occur in close proximity to an epithelial cell of the gingiva, then damage might result. However, activated C8 is generally more efficient in damaging heterologous cells (e.g. bacteria) than host cells.

Immune complex damage: the Arthus reaction
Antigen–antibody complexes in antibody excess occur when relatively small amounts of antigen are introduced into an individual with high titres of circulating antibodies; such a situation could conceivably occur in periodontal disease with the antigen being of bacterial origin. The antigen precipitates with the antibody within or around the vessel wall. Following fixation of complement, PMNL are attracted to the site and accumulate around the blood vessels where they attempt to phagocytose the antigen–antibody complexes. The release of lysosomal enzymes from the PMNL leads to tissue damage. Several attempts have been made to determine whether immune complexes are formed within the tissues in gingivitis and chronic periodontal disease. So far, these attempts have proved to be negative.

Lymphokine production
Activation of lymphocytes within the gingival infiltrate by antigen would lead to lymphokine production. Lymphotoxin may produce non-specific damage in the area to, for example, fibroblasts or osteoblasts. Osteoclast-activating factor, another lymphokine, has been mentioned already (Fig. 3.6).

In the examples quoted above, the normal immune response directed against non-self antigens may, inadvertently, produce damage to the host. The other possible mechanism is that of autoimmunity itself. Autoimmunity is direct reactivity with self antigens. It has been suggested that periodontal disease is an autoimmune disease in which the tissue damage is initiated by antibodies reacting with the patients' own cells. To produce tissue damage, antibodies require the help of accessory mechanisms such as (a) the complement system, (b) phagocytic cells, and (c) K cells. These mechanisms are brought into play after combination of antibody with antigen, the trigger being either a critical alignment of antibody molecules on the antigen surface or a steric change in the Fc part of the bound antibody molecule.

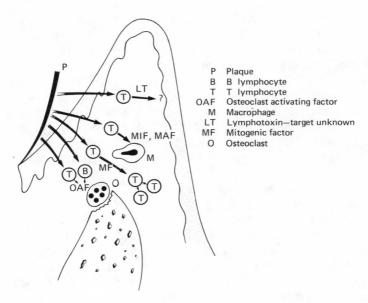

P	Plaque
B	B lymphocyte
T	T lymphocyte
OAF	Osteoclast activating factor
M	Macrophage
LT	Lymphotoxin—target unknown
MF	Mitogenic factor
O	Osteoclast

Fig. 3.6   Soluble factors released by lymphocytes.

(a) Complement activation in this instance would be initiated by the combination of the autoantibody with an antigen resident on the surface of the host cell.

(b) Monocytes and PMNL have receptors (Fc receptors) for the Fc region of IgG 1 and IgG 3 antibodies which enable them to adhere to and phagocytose antibody-coated antigens much more readily than non-complexed antigens. Phagocytes also have receptors for the C3b and C3d activation products of the C3 complement component. This is an efficient way of promoting phagocytosis, as for every antibody molecule bound to an antigen surface many molecules of C3 may be bound.

(c) K (killer) cells have a lymphocyte-like morphology but have cell-surface markers which distinguish them from T and B lymphocytes. Their Fc receptors permit them to bind to the complexed antibodies of all four IgG subclasses. K cells are not phagocytic, when adhering to an IgG antibody-coated cell they can kill the cell by an extracellular mechanism.

Despite the theoretical possibility that autoimmunity is involved in periodontal disease, there is little evidence for the presence of autoantibodies. However, an *in vitro* killing of gingival epithelial cells by peripheral blood lymphocytes from patients with periodontal disease has been recorded and would appear to be an autoimmune mechanism. There is some evidence that T cell cytotoxicity is responsible and that the mechanism may be an *in vitro* demonstration of cross-reactivity between antigens of dental plaque bacteria and of the oral epithelial cell.

Summary

Perhaps the strongest evidence for the role of the specific immune response in the pathogenesis of periodontal disease is provided by the investigation of patients receiving immunosuppressive therapy or those suffering from immunodeficiency. In both groups of patients; the degree of periodontal disease is less than that which might be expected from the amount of dental plaque present. Patients with defective non-specific immunity, that is, PMNL dysfunction, are an exception to this rule in that they have severe periodontal disease (see Chapter 8). In addition, an investigation employing the immunostimulatory drug levamisole showed that an increase in the gingivitis was accompanied by an increase in the cellular immune response to antigens of dental plaque bacteria. It would appear that the presence of dental bacterial plaque, in addition to exerting a direct damaging effect upon the gingiva and periodontium, may also evoke a response on the part of the host which may contribute towards the damage.

Further reading

Ivanyi, L. and Lehner, T. (1977). The effect of Levamisole on gingival inflammation in man. *Scandinavian Journal of Immunology* **6**, 219–26.

Lang, N. P. and Smith F. N. (1976). Lymphocyte response to T-cell mitogen during experimental gingivitis in humans. *Infection and Immunity* **13**, 108–13.

Lehner, T. (1975). Immunological aspects of dental caries and periodontal disease. *British Medical Bulletin* **31**, No. 2, 125–30.

Mackler, B. F., Waldrop, T. C., Schur, P., Robertson, S. E. and Siraganian, R. P. (1978). IgG subclasses in human periodontal disease. I. Distribution and incidence of IgG subclass-bearing lymphocytes and plasma cells. *Journal of Periodontal Research* **13**, 109–19.

Olsson-Wennströöm, A., Wennströöm, J. L., Mergenhagen, S. E. and Siraganian, R. P. (1978). The mechanism of basophil histamine release in patients with periodontal disease. *Clinical and Experimental Immunology* **33**, 166–73.

Page, R. C., Davies, P. and Allison, A. C. (1973). Effects of dental plaque on the production and release of lysosomal hydrolases by macrophages in culture. *Archives of Oral Biology* **18**, 1481–95.

Nisengard, R. J. (1977). The role of immunology in periodontal disease. *Journal of Periodontology* **48**, 505–16.

4

Candidosis

The genus candida comprises a group of unicellular fungi or yeasts. The species *Candida albicans* is responsible for most oral candidal infections or candidosis. The yeast is carried in limited numbers on the oral mucosa as a harmless commensal (in the form of blastospores) in just under 50 per cent of healthy dentate subjects, and in a slightly higher proportion of denture wearers. In the dentate person, candida is isolated most frequently and in greatest numbers from the dorsum of the tongue, which forms the primary oral reservoir for the organism. The cheeks and palate are the other favoured oral sites.

In acute pseudomembranous candidosis, the density of *C. albicans* exceeds the limit observed in health and large numbers of hyphae and spores accumulate in white plaques. The depapillated tongue of acute atrophic candidosis (antibiotic sore mouth) is the hallmark of candidal overgrowth resulting from suppression of the normal bacterial flora by antibiotics (Fig. 4.1).

In chronic hyperplastic candidosis (candidal leukoplakia), a premalignant condition, limited numbers of candidal hyphae penetrate the superficial layers of the epithelium. Candida will also invade the oral epithelium in mucocutaneous candidoses, a rare group of conditions, often genetically determined, but here the oral lesions have no malignant potential.

The structure of *C. albicans*

C. albicans has an outer cell wall essentially composed of glycoproteins, each consisting of branched polysaccharide mannans or glucans (complexed to protein). Variations in the side chains may account for the different antigens detectable in the cell wall. Glycoproteins of the surface layer of the cell wall may bind to specific receptor sites on oral epithelium during candidal colonization. To add to the complexity of the organism, as many as seventy-eight protein antigens have been distinguished within the cytoplasm.

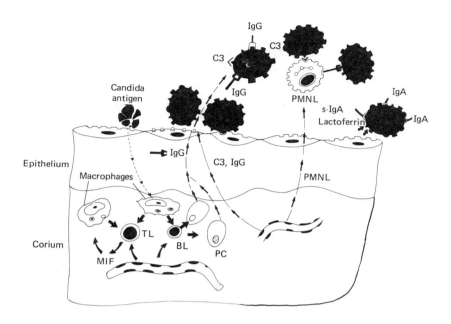

Fig. 4.1 Mucosal defences against candida. The healthy oral epithelium forms a barrier to candida which is continually removed by the flow of saliva containing lactoferrin (which inhibits growth) and specific s-IgA antibody which inhibits adherence of the organism. Candida is opsonized by IgG antibody derived from serum IgG and by activated complement C3, and both factors facilitate phagocytosis by PMNL.

Immunodiagnosis of candidosis

Serum antibodies of the IgG, IgM, IgA and IgE classes are detectable by such techniques as indirect immunofluorescence (see Fig. 1.11). These fluorescent antibody titres are highest in patients with chronic atrophic candidosis (denture stomatitis) and elevated in other forms of oral candidosis. Candidal carriers tend to have lower levels of antibodies than people with overt disease. The diagnosis of superficial candidosis of skin and mucous membranes is easily confirmed with conventional smears and cultures or, in the case of chronic hyperplastic candidosis, by biopsy. What we lack is a reliable serological test for the diagnosis of candidosis in inaccessible sites, such as candidal endocarditis, or in disseminated candidal infections which may be a terminal event in advanced malignancy, particularly when the latter is treated by cytotoxic drugs.

Candidal endocarditis is an extremely grave condition, usually arising from intracardiac surgery or prolonged venous catheterization, but is also associated with drug addiction. Although high or rising titres of serum agglutinins or precipitins to candidal antigens have been demonstrated in patients with endocarditis, similar antibodies can arise after cardiac surgery in uninfected patients. These 'false positive' reactions may be due to increases in the commensal candidal flora in the mouth or other body cavities, particularly during concurrent antibiotic therapy.

The antigenic differences between the mycelial form of candida, associated with tissue invasion, and the blastospore phase, might conceivably form the basis of a serological test to discriminate between invasive and superficial candidosis. Alternatively, the antigen released into the blood in tissue invasion can be detected by sensitive means such as enzyme-linked immunoassays or countercurrent immunoelectrophoresis. Certainly, a rise in serum antibody titre in serial assays on individual patients is more significant than the result of a single estimation.

Defence mechanisms in resistance to oral candidosis (Fig. 4.1)

Whereas, normally, candida cannot be isolated from healthy skin with an intact keratinized epidermis, the yeast may survive on damaged or macerated skin. In addition to this barrier effect, other mechanisms must play a part, as shown by the capacity of the oral mucosa of normal non-carriers to resist colonization after inoculation with candida.

Non-specific mechanisms

Competition from other oral flora
Strept. sanguis, Strept. salivarius and *C. albicans* adhere to oral epithelial cells *in vitro* and can be recovered in substantial numbers from the mucosa of healthy mouths. The oral candidal populations may be limited by bacteria competing with yeasts for specific receptor sites on oral epithelium. Thrush complicating tetracycline therapy may result from unopposed occupation of such receptor sites by candida following elimination of the bacteria by the antibiotic.

Saliva
This flushes the organisms from their oral niches and they are swallowed. Not unexpectedly in xerostomia, oral candidal populations are increased, particularly in the floor of the mouth, where the organisms seldom exist in health due to the usual salivary pool in this region.

In addition to antibody discussed below, saliva contains other substances capable of inhibiting the growth of candida. For example, salivary lactoferrin inhibits growth by complexing the free iron necessary for microbial metabolism.

Phagocytosis
Even when specific opsonizing antibody is absent, PMNL phagocytose and kill candida *in vitro*. A role for PMNL in resistance to oral candidosis is suggested by its frequent occurrence in agranulocytosis or neutropenia. In cases where the agranulocytosis is a complication of cytotoxic therapy for leukaemia or advanced cancer, a fatal disseminated candidosis may be the outcome. In this situation, cell-mediated immunity is also depressed.

Candidosis may also be the mucosal marker of qualitative defects in PMNL function. The cells are either unable to ingest the yeast or, as in chronic granulomatous disease or myeloperoxidase deficiency, intracellular killing is faulty.

Specific defence mechanisms

Antibodies
Agglutinating antibody of secretory IgA type specific for candida can be demonstrated in saliva. The IgA antibody inhibits the adherence of candida to oral epithelium (see Fig. 4.1) and the organisms are removed from the oral cavity during swallowing. However, few patients with defective antibody function (e.g. hypogamma-

globulinaemia or selective IgA deficiency) are susceptible to candidosis. The compensatory production of secretory IgM or IgG, which occurs in some IgA-deficient patients, could be an adequate substitute in defence against candida.

Cell-mediated immunity
The importance of this mechanism is illustrated by patients with either generalized T lymphocyte dysfunction or a selective deficiency of cell-mediated immunity to candida.

C. albicans infections in primary immunodeficiency syndromes

These are congenital or genetically determined disorders in which the children may succumb to overwhelming bacterial or viral infections or malignancy at an early age. Mucocutaneous candidosis may also figure prominently, especially in syndromes where thymic development is abnormal and hence cell-mediated immunity is impaired.

Examples include Di George's syndrome, where both thymus and parathyroid are absent, and severe combined immunodeficiency, an X-lined or autosomal recessive condition, with both failure of thymic development and of antibody formation.

Chronic mucocutaneous candidosis (Tables 4.1–4.4)

In this subgroup, mucocutaneous candidosis forms the major feature and develops in childhood. Usually, children develop oral thrush which becomes persistent, sometimes the condition is genetically determined, often as an autosomal recessive characteristic. Wells and colleagues (1972) delineated four groups on their clinical presentation and mode of inheritance and showed that many of these patients had a defective cellular immune response to candida antigens. Patients with more severe forms of mucocutaneous candidosis have more profound depression of lymphocyte responsiveness to candida antigen. Thus, the more severely affected patients have negative delayed hypersensitivity skin reactions (Table 4.4) to injections of candida extract. *In vitro*, the patients' blood lymphocytes are often not stimulated by candida antigens to divide or to secrete the lymphokine, macrophage migration inhibitory factor (MIF, see Fig. 3.2).

Many patients are iron deficient. Further, in iron deficiency in patients without immune abnormalities one can demonstrate a reduced *in vitro* cell-mediated immune response to candida which

Table 4.1 Classification of oral candidosis. Group I: oral candidosis as part of mucocutaneous candidosis occurring in patients with a profound immune deficiency syndrome. The patients usually die from other diseases and the mucocutaneous candidosis remains superficial and not life threatening. (From Valdimarsson, H. T. (1973). *Cellular Immunology* **6**, 348–61.)

Syndrome	Inheritance	Distribution	Onset	Prognosis
Severe combined immunodeficiency Di George syndrome Chronic granulomatous disease	Congenital or genetically determined	Skin, nails, oral mucosa	Childhood	Usually die from other disease in first few years of life

Table 4.2 Classification of oral candidosis. Group II: chronic mucocutaneous candidosis is the predominant feature but is not fatal, that is, patients do not die from disseminated candidosis. Their candidosis remains superficial. All patients have chronic hyperplastic oral candidosis

Subgroup	Syndrome	Inheritance	Onset	Clinical features, distribution of candidosis
1	Familial chronic mucocutaneous candidosis	Autosomal recessive	Early—before 10 years of age	Mouth, nails, skin; other sites sometimes affected
2	Diffuse chronic mucocutaneous candidosis	Unknown	Early—before 5 years of age	Mouth, skin and nails extensively involved, often with granulomas; eyes, pharynx and larynx; susceptibility to other infection
3	Candida—endocrinopathy	Autosomal recessive	By second decade	Mouth, hypoparathyroidism; hypoadrenocorticism, hypothyroidism and diabetes mellitus
4	Familial mucocutaneous candidosis	Autosomal dominant	In the first year of life	Mouth, nails, scalp, flexures

Table 4.3 Classification of oral candidosis. Group III: this group comprises the common forms of oral candidosis, usually confined to the mouth. The candidosis is usually transient (1) and (2), responds to local treatment and often a local or general predisposing factor is present

Subgroup		Syndrome	Inheritance	Onset	Clinical features
1	Acute	Acute pseudomembranous candidosis (thrush)	None	Any age	Oral mucosa, but can rarely extend to oesophagus; neonates and debilitated adults most commonly
2	Acute	Atrophic candidosis	None	Any age	Transient; follows antibiotic therapy
3	Chronic	Chronic atrophic	None	Any age	'Denture sore mouth'; usually confined to denture-bearing area of mucosa; reversible on removing denture or appliance
4	Chronic	Chronic hyperplastic candidosis	None	After age 30	Premalignant oral white plaques

Table 4.4 Tests of cell-mediated immunity in chronic mucocutaneous candidosis with immune defects Grade I (most severe) to IV (no defect detected) (By courtesy of Dr H. Valdimarsson and *Cellular Immunology*.)

	Lymphocyte transformation	Candida inhibitory factor present in serum	MIF production	Skin testing for delayed hypersensitivity Candida	PPD	DNCB
I	+	−	−	−	−	−
II	−	−	+	−	−	−
III	−	+	−	−	−	−
IV	+	−	+	+	+	+

PPD, purified protein derivative (*Mycobacterium tuberculosis*); DNCB, dinitrochlorobenzene (See Fig. 2.7); MIF, macrophage inhibitory factor.
+, normal; −, absent.

returns to normal when iron therapy is administered. Consistent with this, when iron-deficient patients with chronic mucocutaneous candidiasis receive iron therapy, the candidosis improves but is not cured.

However, patients with chronic mucocutaneous candidosis have normal levels of candidal antibody in their blood and saliva. The miscellaneous reports of serum inhibitors to leucocyte phagocytosis and killing of candida, abnormal macrophage function, complement defects and autoantibody production serve to illustrate the complexity of the problem.

Patients with chronic mucocutaneous candidosis have an inherited lack of T lymphocytes capable of responding to candida and additionally to other antigens in severe cases. Grafts of thymus or cell-free extracts of thymus (thymosin) have been used to restore to normal immune responses in patients with chronic mucocutaneous candidiasis associated with a wide-ranging T cell dysfunction. For subjects with a selective immune deficiency in response to candida alone, blood leucocytes from siblings or a cell-free extract of the leucocytes (transfer factor) have been employed. As a result of this immunological rehabilitation, a number of patients have enjoyed a dramatic improvement in their candidosis, although sometimes the benefit has only been temporary. Grafting of viable cells to patients with a more profound immunodysfunction runs the risk of a serious or fatal graft-versus-host reaction in which the transferred cells recognize the host as foreign, and the histocompatibility antigens of host and donor should ideally be perfectly matched.

Reference

Wells, R. S., Higgs, J. M., Macdonald, A., Valdimarsson, H. and Holt, P. J. L. (1972). Familial chronic mucocutaneous candidiasis. *Journal of Medical Genetics* **9**, 302–310.

Further reading

Arendorf, T. M. and Walker, D. M. (1980). The prevalence and intra-oral distribution of *Candida albicans* in man. *Archives of Oral Biology* **25**, 1–10.

Cawson, R. A. (1966). Chronic oral candidiasis and leukoplakia. *Oral Surgery* **22**, 582–91.

Higgs, J. M. and Wells, R. S. (1973). Chronic mucocutaneous candidiasis, new approaches to treatment. *British Journal of Dermatology* **89**, 179–90.

Lehner, T. (1966). Immunofluorescent study of *Candida albicans* in candidiasis, carriers and controls. *Journal of Pathology and Bacteriology* **91**, 97–104.

Lehner, T., Wilton, J. M. and Ivanyi, L. (1972). Immunodeficiencies in chronic mucocutaneous candidosis. *Immunology* **22**, 775–87.

Valdimarsson, H., Higgs, J. M., Yamamura, M., Hobbs, J. R. and Holt, P. J. L. (1973). Immune abnormalities associated with chronic mucocutaneous candidiasis. *Cellular Immunology* **6**, 348–61.

Walker, D. M. (1975). Candidal infection of the oral mucosa. In *The oral mucosa in health and disease*, pp. 467–505. Ed. by A. E. Dolby. Blackwell, Oxford.

5

Viral Infections

Viral infections of the mouth are most frequently due to the herpes simplex virus, but occasionally herpes zoster affecting the trigeminal nerve may involve the oral mucosa. Hand, foot and mouth disease, and herpangina are uncommon oral vesicular eruptions caused by viruses of the Coxsackie A group.

Herpes simplex

The herpes virus hominis type I has a central DNA core, surrounded by a protein shell or capsid consisting of 162 capsomeres (protein subunits) arranged to form a symmetrical icosahedron. Outside this there is a lipoprotein cell envelope containing host cell-derived material.

To initiate an infection, the virus adsorbs to the host cell surface which it then penetrates, leaving behind its cell envelope. The virus then replicates intracellularly and subsequently virus-specific antigens appear on the membrane of the infected cell. The virus spreads from cell to cell within the epithelium via intercellular junctions. The infected cells become swollen and oedematous, the cell membranes degenerate, the cells coalesce and a vesicle forms.

Acute gingivostomatitis

Primary infection with herpes simplex type I usually occurs in childhood or adolescence, presenting as a vesicular eruption in the oral mucosa with enlargement of the gingivae. Recurrence of the infection in the mouth is very rare although, as discussed below, after this primary infection the virus can persist in a latent form and may subsequently cause recurrent lesions at extra-oral sites.

Seven to ten days after the onset of the acute gingivostomatitis there is a diagnostic rise in the serum titre of antibody, as measured by viral neutralization and complement-fixation techniques. Initially, the virus-specific antibody is of the IgM class and its appearance is followed by a rise in IgG antibody. The antibodies are directed against antigens of the protein shell and cell envelope. According to serum antibody determination, most of the population have had a primary herpes simplex infection by the time they reach adolescence and it seems that many of these infections are silent or go unrecognized. Recovery correlates not only with the rise in antibody titre but also with the presence in peripheral blood of lymphocytes which release MIF on contact with herpes antigens.

Antibody-mediated immunity (Fig. 5.1)

Antibodies can prevent the spread of virus in two ways. Firstly, antibody interacting with the free virus could 'neutralize' it by masking its receptors for oral epithelial cells (Fig. 5.1a). Secondly,

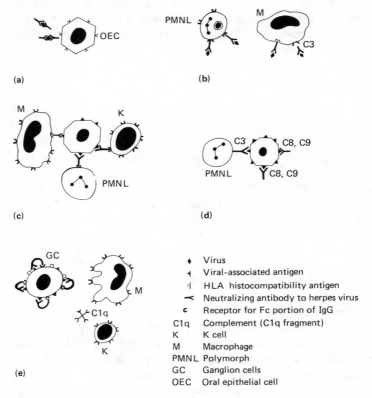

Fig. 5.1   Antibody-mediated immunity in herpes simplex infection. **(a)** Neutralizing antibody blocks binding sites of virus for oral epithelial cells. **(b)** Antibody and complement (C3) promote phagocytosis of virus by polymorph or macrophage. **(c)** Killing of virus-infected epithelial cell via the Fc receptor for IgG antibody by phagocytosis (polymorphs or macrophages) or by K cells. **(d)** Direct killing of virus-infected cell. C8, C9 complement components activated by antibody or indirectly by phagocytosis via the C3 receptor. **(e)** Mechanisms by which herpes simplex virus remain latent in trigeminal ganglion cells.

virus–antibody complexes could be phagocytosed by macrophages or PMNL and the virus degraded intracellularly (Fig. 5.1b). Opsonization may be mediated via the C3 receptor if the virus–antibody complex activates complement, or through the Fc receptor if the antibody is of the IgG class.

Antibodies are also potentially capable of killing virus-infected cells by binding to the virus-determined antigen on the cell surface, and triggering one or more of the accessory mechanisms, as discussed below.

1. If the antibody is of the IgG class, phagocytic cells may attempt to phagocytose the virus-infected cell via the Fc receptor. There is another cell type, known as K (for killer) cells which also have Fc receptors (Fig. 5.1c). K cells are non-phagocytic cells which kill their target cells by an extracellular mechanism requiring intimate cell contact. Morphologically, K cells have the appearance of large granular lymphocytes and have many properties in common with NK cells.

2. If the antibody can activate complement, complement-derived chemotactic factors will attract phagocytic cells and phagocytosis can proceed via the C3 receptor (Fig. 5.1d).

3. Even in the absence of phagocytic cells, complement activation can led to death of the virus-infected cell due to cell membrane damage by the C8 and C9 complement components (Fig. 5.1d). Surprisingly, in this situation with IgG antibodies, complement is activated not as expected by the classical pathway but by the alternative pathway. This also seems to be true for lysis of cells infected with a number of other viruses.

Mechanisms by which herpes-infected cells avoid attack by antibodies

Despite the impressive array of effector mechanisms which can be triggered by antibody, cell-mediated immunity seems to be of prime importance, as discussed below. Two observations may explain the relative ineffectiveness of antibody in eliminating herpes virus-infected cells.

1. If antibody is present in small amounts, sufficient to activate complement only to a small extent or not at all, the virus antigen–antibody complexes on the membrane of an infected cell migrate to and coalesce at one pole of the cell. This phenomenon is known as capping. The capped complexes are then shed from the cell, leaving the cell membrane of the infected cell free of virus-determined

antigens and hence resistant to further attack by antibody or cytotoxic T cells. Such cells could then serve as a source of infection for neighbouring cells.

2. Normally, only certain cell types of the lymphoid or myeloid series have receptors for the Fc portion of IgG antibodies. However, other cell types can acquire Fc receptors after infection with herpes viruses. (Are they cell or virus-coded?) If antibody binds to virus-determined antigen on the membrane of the infected cell, then the Fc portion of the molecule may be bound by an adjacent Fc receptor on the same cell and hence be sequestered from the Fc receptors of phagocytic cells and K cells and from the C1 component of complement (Fig. 5.1e). There is some data to suggest that if the Fc receptors of herpes-infected cells are occupied in this way then viral replication is inhibited. This could provide an explanation for the phenomena of 'latency' (see recurrent herpes simplex infections).

Cell-mediated immunity

As mentioned above, recovery from primary herpetic gingivostomatitis correlates with MIF production by lymphocytes. This is usually taken as a manifestation of cellular immunity, although it is now recognized that B lymphocytes as well as T cells can produce MIF.

Production of MIF and other lymphokines at the site of infection will attract macrophages which even in the absence of antibody have a limited capacity to ingest and kill herpes simplex viruses. As well as immobilizing macrophages, MIF increases their viricidal activity.

Presumably also present at the infection site are specific cytotoxic T lymphocytes—these are readily detected by *in vitro* assays but less easy to demonstrate *in vivo*. The cytotoxic T cells recognize the virus-determined antigen on the membrane of the infected cells. In particular they appear to recognize a complex of virus-determined antigen and the cell's HLA transplantation antigens (Fig. 5.2). This is deduced from the observation that cytotoxic T cells will only kill virus-infected cells of the same HLA phenotype as themselves (this restriction is true in most of the virus–cytotoxic T cell combinations tested). As a result of this direct interaction between cytotoxic T cells and virus-infected target cell, the latter is killed—again close apposition of killer and target cell is required. Virus is liberated into the extracellular space where it is more amenable to immunological attack.

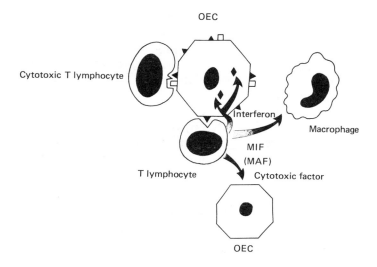

OEC   Oral epithelial cell
MIF   Migration inhibitory factor
⊏╵   HLA histocompatibility antigen
◀   Viral–associated antigen
MAF   Macrophage activating factor

Fig. 5.2   Cell-mediated immunity in herpes simplex infection.

Interferon

Interferon is one of the lymphokines produced after specific T lymphocytes interact with herpes antigens. Interferons are a family of glycoproteins of molecular weight 13 000–26 000 which have antiviral activity. Most types of virus are susceptible, although in general RNA viruses are more susceptible than DNA viruses. Interferons have no direct effect on viruses but act by inhibiting viral replication in infected cells by preventing translation of virus messenger RNA (Fig. 5.2). They also have a range of other biological effects, including controlling the growth and differentiation of certain cell types such as lymphoid cells. The interferon produced by T lymphocytes on antigenic stimulation (termed γ-interferon) differs physicochemically and functionally from other interferons, although it shares their antiviral activity. Interferons produced by other cell types (termed α-and β-interferons) are synthesized as a result of virus infection. As viral replication is well under way in the infected cells, interferon production has no effect on the fate of the parent cell, but its release and uptake by neighbouring uninfected cells can help protect these from viral infection. In fact, interferon production early in virus infection is an important non-specific defence mechanism limiting spread of the infection until such time as the specific immune mechanisms can come into play.

Although in *in vitro* assays replication of herpes simplex virus is only marginally inhibited by interferon, the effect *in vivo* is much more dramatic. This suggests that the effects of interferon on the immune system may be at least as important in terms of antiviral resistance as its direct effects on viral replication.

Recurrent herpes simplex infection

In up to half the general population, the virus is not completely eliminated after the primary infection. It resides, latent, in the sensory ganglion of the trigeminal nerve, effectively sequestered from the immune system yet apparently not harming the surrounding neurons. It is not yet clear why the virus homes to this site, although it may remain there for many years without replication. Viral replication may be subsequently triggered by respiratory tract infections, fevers or menstruation. The viruses travel down the axons of the sensory nerves to nerve endings on the lips or elsewhere on the face where a vesicular eruption or 'cold sore' results. Individuals subject to this recurrent herpes labialis have adequate or even high levels of antibody in their blood. Their cellular responses to herpes hominis virus I tend to be subnormal in *in vitro* tests of lymphocyte function, such as lymphocyte transformation and particularly macrophage migration inhibitory factor production. The impaired cell-mediated immune response, probably due to incompetent T lymphocytes, apparently underlies this susceptibility to such recurrent viral infections. Recurrent cold sores affect a significant proportion of the population and the T cell defect appears to be restricted to herpes antigens; affected individuals do not have severe infections with other micro-organisms.

Summary

There is evidence that both antibody and cell-mediated immunity have roles to play. Neonatal herpetic gingivostomatitis is rare, due perhaps to the passive transfer of maternal antibody. Further recurrent intra-oral infections with herpes simplex type I are very uncommon and it could be postulated that neutralizing secretory IgA antibodies can account for this. On the other hand, patients with hypogammaglobulinaemia do not have an especially severe form of gingivostomatitis, nor are they susceptible to repeated attacks in this site. Patients with impaired cell-mediated immunity do have serious problems, indicating that cell-mediated immunity is probably of prime importance, with antibody-mediated mechanisms playing a supporting role.

Further reading

Gibbs, C. G., Nemo, G. J. and Diwan, A. R. (1979). Immunology of persistent and recurrent viral infections. In *Immunological Aspects of Infectious Disease*, pp. 462–7. Ed. by G. Dick. MTP Press, Lancaster.

Nahmias, A. J., Shore, S. L., Kohl, S., Starr, S. E. and Ashman, R. B. (1976). Immunology of herpes simplex virus infection. Relevance to herpes simplex virus vaccines and cervical cancer. *Cancer Research* **36**, 836–44.

Notkins, A. L. (Ed.) (1975). *Viral immunology and immunopathology*. Academic Press, New York.

6

Ulcerative and Bullous Lesions

Recurrent oral ulceration

The clinical diagnosis of recurrent oral ulceration encompasses several quite different diseases, in each of which the immunological events may be of aetiological significance.

Recurrent aphthous ulceration

In the initial stages of the disease process the basal and spinous layers of the oral epithelium are infiltrated by small mononuclear cells and there is coincident destruction of the epithelium. With the onset of ulceration there is an influx of PMNLs. Immunofluorescent studies have revealed the presence of C3 in vessel walls and in the subepithelial zone of the ulcers (Fig. 6.1).

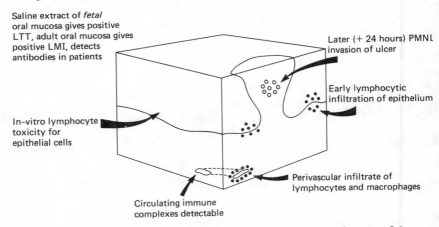

Saline extract of *fetal* oral mucosa gives positive LTT, adult oral mucosa gives positive LMI, detects antibodies in patients

Later (+ 24 hours) PMNL invasion of ulcer

Early lymphocytic infiltration of epithelium

In-vitro lymphocyte toxicity for epithelial cells

Perivascular infiltrate of lymphocytes and macrophages

Circulating immune complexes detectable

Fig. 6.1 Aphthous ulceration: abnormalities detectable (left) and features of the ulcer (right). LTT, lymphocyte transformation test (see Fig. 3.3); LMI, leucocyte migration inhibition (see Fig. 3.2).

The following immunological abnormalities have been detected in many of the patients.

1. Elevated antibody titres (IgG + IgM) to a saline extract of fetal

72

oral mucosa, detected by agglutination and precipitation reactions. The titres were higher than in subjects with oral ulceration from other causes.

2. Increased lymphocyte transformation (see Fig. 3.3) with a saline extract of fetal oral mucosa. In a sequential study the increase correlated with disease activity.

3. Inhibition of leucocyte migration (see Fig. 3.2) with an extract of adult oral mucosa.

4. Cytotoxicity of peripheral blood leucocytes for adult oral epithelial cells in tissue culture.

5. Approximately half of the patients have elevated levels of circulating IgG immune complexes, detected by their inhibition of the agglutination of IgG-coated particles by a rabbit IgM antibody to human IgG.

The elevated levels of autoantibody to fetal oral mucosa may arise secondarily because of damage to the oral mucosa, although why the titre of antibody should be higher than in other oral ulcerative diseases is not clear. The increased lymphocyte transformation, leucocyte migration inhibition and detection of lymphocyte toxicity may reflect a cellular immune response to oral epithelial cell antigens. The antigen or antigens, although present in oral epithelium, may not have initiated the humoral and cellular immune response. Instead, the response could have been evoked by a bacterial or viral antigen with a similar antigenic structure to that of the epithelial cell antigen, in the same way as autoantibody reactive with cardiac muscle in rheumatic heart disease may in fact have been induced by streptococcal antigen. *Strept. sanguis* type 2A has been implicated as an organism which may be responsible for this cross-reacting autoimmunity. Levels of serum antibodies to *Strept. sanguis* increase and remain elevated during the course of the ulceration. Patients with the disease respond to intradermal injections of vaccine prepared from the organism by reactions of the 'delayed hypersensitivity' type (see Fig. 2.7). Studies of the cell-mediated immune response *in vitro* to the same organism have been made and have led to contradictory findings. Initial studies showing no lymphocyte transformation with extracts of *Strept. sanguis* in patients suffering from the disease have not been confirmed in recent studies where a larger range of antigen doses has been used. Thus, although cross-reactivity with antigens of an infecting organism offers an attractive explanation for the aetiology of the disease, the existence of such a culpable micro-organism is still uncertain. There is a familial pattern to the disease, which, despite careful study, has not shown any clear hereditary pattern.

Behçet's syndrome

Recurrent oral ulceration is an almost invariable symptom in this disease, the immunological aspects of which are reminiscent of recurrent aphthous ulceration. Unfortunately, there is no *in vitro* diagnostic test which serves to distinguish between the patient with the painful but innocuous recurrent oral aphthae and Behçet's syndrome. Thus, there is similar evidence of elevated levels of antibody to fetal oral mucosa and it has been suggested that the greater incidence of immune complexes in Behçet's syndrome may account for the ulceration of skin and genitalia and the involvement of the central nervous system. With such pronounced vascular damage in the lesions, it would be expected that the oral ulcers in Behçet's syndrome would be severe, more akin to the major variety of recurrent aphthae than the minor variety. Although this is very often the case, it is not always so, both minor aphthae and the rare herpetiform pattern of recurrent oral ulceration are also found. The latter form of recurrent oral ulceration, despite a similar clinical appearance to the intra-oral type I herpetic infection, is apparently not caused by that virus and similar immunological abnormalities are found as in recurrent oral aphthae. A search for a viral aetiology in recurrent oral aphthae and Behçet's syndrome has so far been unsuccessful. In Behçet's syndrome, recourse has often to be made to anti-inflammatory, immunosuppressive drugs, but none of the *in vitro* immunological phenomena relating to the disease has proved to be of value in either monitoring the disease or in distinguishing the more severe Behçet's syndrome from recurrent oral ulceration.

In Behçet's syndrome there is, as with recurrent aphthous ulceration, a familial predisposition to the disease. In recent years, attempts have been made to relate the incidence of the disease to genetic markers, especially transplantation antigens.

Transplantation antigens are coded at four main loci—HLA (human leucocyte antigen)-A, -B, -C and -D on chromosome 6. There are many possible alleles at each locus (e.g. more than 20 at the HLA-A locus) and these are inherited in Mendelian fashion (Fig. 6.2). The HLA-A, B and C antigens are present in highest amounts on leucocytes but are present also on many other cell types, HLA-D antigens are confined to certain cells (e.g. lymphocytes, macrophages, epithelial cells). Typing for HLA-A, B and C transplantation antigens is done by a serological method, employing complement-dependent cytotoxicity in the presence of specific anti-HLA sera. These sera are obtained from multiparous women or from patients who have had multiple blood transfusions. Serological methods for HLA-D typing are now becoming available to replace the cumbersome method of mixed lymphocyte reactivity. This relies upon the fact that when lymphocyte populations with different HLA-D antigens are mixed, they recognize the alien HLA-D antigens and divide. This method takes four to five days to perform and is quantitated by

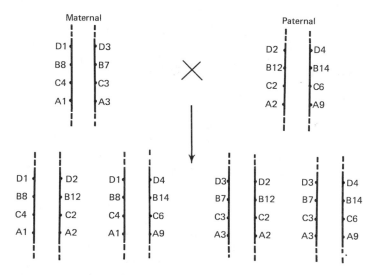

Fig. 6.2 Mendelian inheritance of transplantation antigens. The antigens are coded at four loci on chromosome 6 and the alleles at each locus are designated by number, e.g. D1, D2, D3 etc. The offspring of the pairing above can have one of four combinations of HLA antigens (as each maternal chromosome 6 can be paired with either of the paternal chromosome 6's).

measuring the uptake of ^{3}H-thymidine into DNA. The drawback is that the test takes four to five days and necessitates the storage of a representative panel of lymphocytes in liquid nitrogen.

Several diseases have been shown to have a relationship to the HLA characteristics of the individuals and in Behçet's syndrome a high prevalence of HLA-B5 has been recorded in studies in Japan and the Middle East, this has not been observed in the United Kingdom and USA. However, a recent United Kingdom study found that different subtypes of Behçet's syndrome were associated with HLA antigen, HLA-B5 with the ocular type, HLA-B27 with the arthritic type and HLA-B12 with the mucocutaneous type.

The oral ulcers in Behçet's syndrome, as in recurrent aphthous ulceration, are characterized histologically by a PMNL infiltrate from twenty-four hours onwards. Serum from Behçet's patients has increased chemotactic capacity and, although this is not unique to the disease, the PMNL do have an abnormally high response to a chemotactic stimulus.

Ulcerative colitis

In addition to the fact that recurrent oral ulcers occur commonly in this disease, there is an interesting parallel with the immunological abnormalities of recurrent aphthous ulceration. Thus, there is an elevated titre of antibody and cell-mediated reactivity to fetal colon. A similar search for a bacterium with antigenic cross-reacting characteristics with colon (as for mucosa in recurrent aphthae) has led to the discovery that *Esch. coli 0014* does indeed have antigenic characteristics which cross-react with colonic tissue. The reason for the association of oral aphthae and ulcerative colitis is unknown. It does not seem to be due to reactivity against common antigens in the mucosa of the mouth and the gut.

Coeliac disease

Again, oral ulcers indistinguishable from recurrent aphthae occur commonly in this disease, which is due apparently to an indirect effect of a toxic component of gluten acting on the small intestinal epithelium. Conversely, coeliac disease has been claimed to be more common in patients with recurrent aphthae, although this observation has been disputed in further studies. A number of immunological mechanisms have been implicated in the atrophy of the small intestine in coeliac disease. The association of the two diseases remains unexplained and the possible effect of a diet free of gluten on the course of recurrent aphthous ulceration has been examined to only a limited extent and requires further study.

Bullous lesions

Pemphigus and bullous pemphigoid

These two groups of disease are, in general, characterized immunologically by antibodies against anatomical sites which are related to the histology of the lesion. Thus in pemphigus, histological examination of the bullous lesions reveals them to be intraepithelial bullae, which tend to rupture easily and are apparently caused by loss of cohesion between epithelial cells. The antibody in pemphigus is IgG or IgM directed against the intercellular cement substance of the epithelial cells (Fig. 6.3). In pemphigoid, the large, tense blisters are subepidermal bullae and the antibody is directed against the basement membrane zone (Fig. 6.4). Both antibodies may be detected by the fluorescent antibody technique (see Fig. 1.11). In pemphigus, since the titre of antibody to intercellular material tends to rise prior to an exacerbation of the disease and fall before an improvement, the measurement of the titre is an aid in management. In addition, this

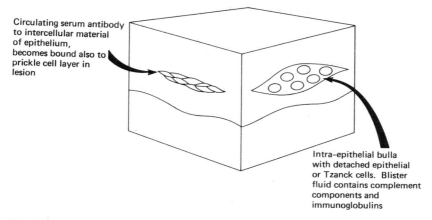

Circulating serum antibody to intercellular material of epithelium, becomes bound also to prickle cell layer in lesion

Intra-epithelial bulla with detached epithelial or Tzanck cells. Blister fluid contains complement components and immunoglobulins

Fig. 6.3 Pemphigus: site of lesion and immunological abnormalities.

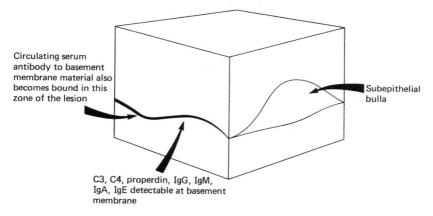

Circulating serum antibody to basement membrane material also becomes bound in this zone of the lesion

Subepithelial bulla

C3, C4, properdin, IgG, IgM, IgA, IgE detectable at basement membrane

Fig. 6.4 Bullous pemphigoid: site of lesion and immunological abnormalities.

fact has been put forward as evidence for the pathological role of antibody in the disease. Drugs, such as cortisone and azathiaprine, which in addition to other effects reduce the titre of antibody, lead to improvement in the disease. In addition, plasmapheresis—that is, replacement of the patient's plasma with that from a normal subject—often leads to temporary remission. Alternatively, the antibody may reflect tissue damage occurring as a result of the disease process as a similar antibody is found after severe burns. The interaction of antigen and antibody may lead to activation of complement at the site and complement components have been detected in the same intercellular areas as immunoglobulin. An alternative explanation is that the autoantibodies may be directed against the cell membrane attachment sites, they may competitively displace the normal cell adhesion bonds.

In pemphigoid there is a poor correlation between the titre of antibody and the disease state, so that the measurement of the titre is not of such great therapeutic value as it is in pemphigus. In addition to immunoglobulin, both classical and alternative complement pathway components have been detected in the basement membrane zone.

A disease with the characteristics of pemphigus, and associated with an arthropod-borne virus infection, occurs in Brazil. The immunological abnormalities are similar and the existence of this disease does raise the possibility that pemphigus found elsewhere in the world may also be due to an immune response against an infecting organism, cross-reacting with epithelial tissue.

Benign mucous membrane pemphigoid

In benign mucous membrane pemphigoid (cicatricial pemphigoid), the circulating antibody to basement membrane material is not detectable, but biopsies of tissue near lesions reveal that immunoglobulin is bound *in vivo* (Fig. 6.5).

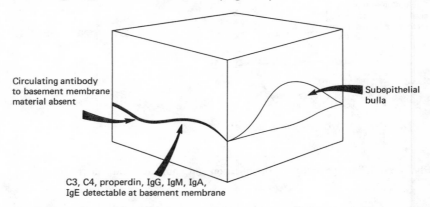

Circulating antibody to basement membrane material absent

Subepithelial bulla

C3, C4, properdin, IgG, IgM, IgA, IgE detectable at basement membrane

Fig. 6.5   Benign mucous membrane pemphigoid.

It should be emphasized that benign mucous membrane pemphigoid is the variety of pemphigoid which will be seen most by the dental surgeon; both forms are rare.

Lichen planus

Although several features of this dermatological disease with oral manifestations strongly suggest an immunological basis, the evidence is actually tenuous and circumstantial. The oral lesions may be in the form of white raised plaques, termed 'hypertrophic' lichen planus, or as superficial ulcerative areas, termed the atrophic lesions of lichen planus. There is a pronounced mononuclear infiltrate of the corium underlying the epithelium and this infiltrate in both the oral mucosa and the skin is composed predominantly of T lymphocytes and some macrophages. Colloid bodies, or Civatte bodies, which are seen with routine histology are eosinophilic bodies representing the damaged epithelial cells. Cytoid bodies represent accumulations of IgM at the junction of epithelium and connective tissue and within the connective tissue itself. The cytoid bodies are seen in many other diseases. In addition to the IgM accumulations, small, lesser deposits of IgG, IgA, C3 and C4 are found at the junction of epithelium and connective tissue or within the connective tissue immediately underlying the affected epithelium. There are no circulating autoantibodies (Fig. 6.6).

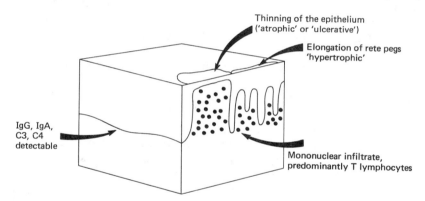

Fig. 6.6 The immunopathology of lichen planus.

In lichen planus, bullae may form from the liquefaction degeneration of the epithelial basal cells, and the immunofluorescent findings in this disease and in pemphigoid may serve to distinguish between those cases where confusion may exist.

Further reading

Beutner, E. H., Chorzelski, T. P., Bean, S. F. (1979). *Immunopathology of the skin: labelled antibody studies*, 2nd edn. John Wiley, New York.
Lehner, T. (1979). *Behçet's syndrome. Clinical and immunological features.* Academic Press, London.

7

Immunity and Neoplasia

In his hypothesis of immunological surveillance, Burnet (1965) suggested that malignant cells arise as a result of a somatic mutation. He postulated that tumour antigens (neoantigens) expressed on the malignant cells are then recognized as 'non-self' by the immune system which proceeds to destroy the abnormal cells. If Burnet's hypothesis is correct:

(i) clinically overt cancers must be either non-antigenic or, alternatively, they are antigenic but somehow avoid surveillance;

(ii) Malignancy should occur with increased frequency in an immunodeficient population.

Many studies of tumour immunology have now shown that various types of cancer cell have antigens not present on normal cells of that type and that these tumours grow because the immune response of the host is inadequate. However, most of these data have been gleaned from studies in experimental animals with transplantable tumours, rather than with tumours arising spontaneously which offer better models for human cancer. In fact, spontaneous tumours in animals turn out not to be antigenic.

There is indisputably a greater incidence of malignancy in immunosuppressed individuals compared with that in normal subjects, but the neoplasms are lymphomas, leukaemias and certain types of skin cancer rather than the commoner types of cancers of the lung, breast, stomach or colon. The high incidence of lymphoid neoplasms is probably more readily explicable by the high mitotic rate of the residual lymphoid tissue with a correspondingly greater risk of mutation, be it spontaneous or induced by carcinogen or virus.

There are a number of problems involved in studying the immunology of neoplasia. Firstly, many experiments designed to study tumour antigens can only be performed in experimental animals. Secondly, it is much easier to use transplantable animal tumours which do not have the experimental drawbacks of arising unpredictably in a small proportion of the animal colony. Thirdly, when *in vitro* studies are employed, either with human or animal systems, the cancer cells used have been adapted to grow continuously in tissue culture and may not be representative of the original cancer cell population.

Because of these problems, much of the evidence discussed below may not be directly relevant to human cancer.

Detection of tumour antigens by in vivo tests

The simplest approach is to excise a locally growing tumour, make a suspension of the tumour cells and reinject some of these into a different site in the same animal. If the tumour is antigenic, then the injected cells will be rejected, if it is not antigenic, then the tumour will grow again at the injection site. An alternative method is to inject an animal with tumour cells from a syngeneic (genetically identical) animal. The injected tumour cells would have been previously treated with mitomycin C or x-rays to inhibit cell division. After one or more injections, in an attempt to stimulate the immune response, the animal is challenged with viable tumour cells. If the tumour is antigenic it will be rejected, if not it will grow.

Such studies have shown that tumours induced by oncogenic viruses are frequently antigenic, as are those induced by high doses of carcinogens. Tumours induced by low doses of carcinogens or which arise spontaneously are poorly antigenic. A large-scale study over many years of spontaneously arising tumours in an animal breeding centre found that none was antigenic.

Detection of tumour antigens by in vitro tests

In principle, this involves testing sera or lymphoid cells from tumour-bearing hosts for reactivity with intact tumour cells or their extracts using in-vitro techniques. As a negative control, the tests should include normal cells of the same cell type as the tumour cells. These studies are most readily interpretable when tumours from syngeneic animals are employed, as any immune response will be restricted to new antigens on the tumour cells. Nevertheless, more convincing evidence of the presence of tumour antigen can often be obtained by immunizing hosts which are allogeneic (of the same species but genetically dissimilar) or xenogeneic (i.e. of another species). Here, tumour rejection readily occurs because the host 'sees' other antigens on the tumour cell (e.g. transplantation antigens, blood group antigens) in addition to the tumour antigens. The presentation of the tumour antigen in association with the other antigens results in a much stronger host response than would be obtained in a syngeneic system.

Recently, monoclonal antibodies from hybridomas have been used to study tumour antigens (Fig. 7.1). This technique involves taking antibody-producing spleen cells from an animal immunized against the tumour and fusing these with myeloma cells, employing polyethylene glycol (PEG) as the fusing agent. The PEG acts by disrupting the cell membranes. On removal of the PEG, the cell membranes reform whereupon a spleen cell and a myeloma cell may fuse. Unfused myeloma cells lack the purine salvage enzyme

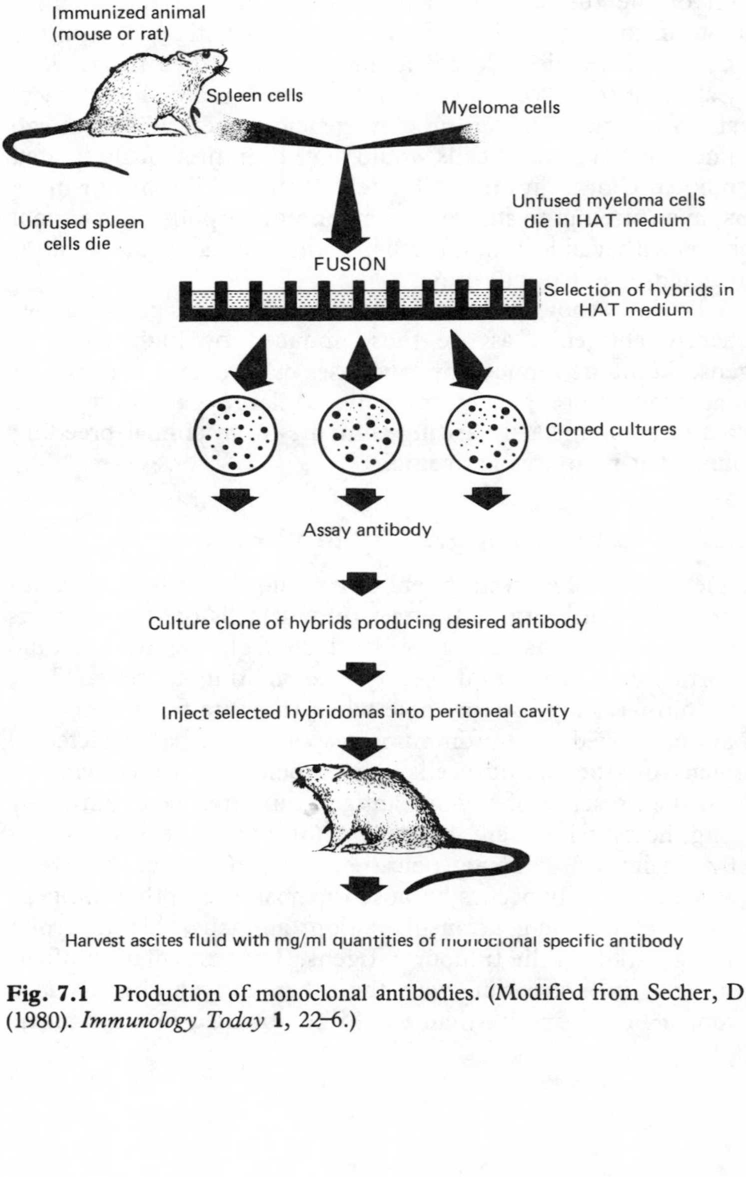

Immunized animal
(mouse or rat)

Spleen cells

Myeloma cells

Unfused spleen
cells die

Unfused myeloma cells
die in HAT medium

FUSION

Selection of hybrids in
HAT medium

Cloned cultures

Assay antibody

Culture clone of hybrids producing desired antibody

Inject selected hybridomas into peritoneal cavity

Harvest ascites fluid with mg/ml quantities of monoclonal specific antibody

Fig. 7.1 Production of monoclonal antibodies. (Modified from Secher, D. S. (1980). *Immunology Today* **1**, 22–6.)

hypoxanthine phosphoribosyl transferase (HPRT) and thus die in a selective medium containing hypoxanthanine, aminopterin and thymidine (HAT). Unfused spleen cells die naturally. Only the hybrid cells survive because they have both the ability to make the HPRT enzyme (inherited from the antibody-producing parent spleen cell) and the potential for unlimited growth of the parent myeloma cell. The surviving hybrid cells are cloned and screened for the production of appropriate antibody. As each cell in the clone is a progeny of a single hybrid precursor, the antibodies are of uniform specificity, i.e. monoclonal. Using this technique it has been shown, for example, that malignant melanoma cells from different patients have antigens in common which normal melanocytes lack.

The nature of tumour antigens

There are three main types.

1. Tumour specific—for example, fibrosarcomas induced by the same chemical carcinogen in corresponding sites in two syngeneic animals have different antigens. Indeed, the same carcinogen injected in multiple sites in one animal can result in several tumours, each with distinct tumour antigens.

2. Tumour associated—these include oncofetal antigens, for example carcinoembryonic antigen (CEA) which can be detected in carcinoma of the colon and which is a differentiation antigen present in normal colonic epithelial cells of the fetus but not the adult. The re-expression in colonic carcinoma cells may be due to uncovering of buried membrane components or to the derepression of the gene coding for CEA.

3. Virally determined—Burkitt's lymphoma tumours induced by an oncogenic virus, the Epstein–Barr virus, all have EB viral antigens.

Paradoxically, normal tissue antigens may be deleted in malignant states. Partial or complete loss of blood group antigens A and B normally present on oral epithelium can occur in premalignant leukoplakia or oral cancer.

A number of carcinogen- or virus-induced tumour antigens have been characterized as glycoprotein, protein or even lipid, in some cases the antigen appears to be linked to the cell's transplantation antigens.

Mechanisms of antitumour immunity

Most information has been derived from *in vitro* assays and therefore needs confirmation in suitably designed *in vivo* tests.

Antibody-mediated mechanism

Antitumour antibody in the presence of complement is often cytotoxic, although a xenogeneic source of complement is usually best, casting some doubt on the efficacy of this mechanism *in vivo* (Fig. 7.2b). In some systems, antibody alone, although not cytotoxic, inhibits tumour growth (Fig. 7.2a). Even non-complement fixing antibody can effectively kill tumour cells in the presence of K cells (Fig. 7.2c).

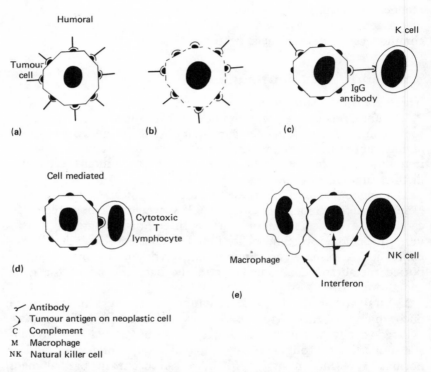

Humoral

Tumour cell

(a)   (b)

K cell

IgG antibody

(c)

Cell mediated

Cytotoxic T lymphocyte

(d)

Macrophage

NK cell

Interferon

(e)

⌐ Antibody
⟩ Tumour antigen on neoplastic cell
C Complement
M Macrophage
NK Natural killer cell

Fig. 7.2   Possible mechanisms in antitumour immunity. **(a)** Growth and spread restricted by antibody. **(b)** Complement-dependent lysis. **(c)** Antibody-dependent cell-mediated cytotoxicity **(d)** Killing by T lymphocyte. **(e)** Killing by macrophages and NK cells.

Cell-mediated immunity

In many models, cell-mediated immunity appears to be of critical importance. Presumably the tumour-reactive T lymphocytes release lymphokines to enlist macrophages in helping them kill the tumour cells or, as described in many *in vitro* systems, the T lymphocytes are directly cytotoxic to the tumour cells (Fig. 7.2d). Often the sera of tumour-bearing animals contain factors which can prevent the action of the cytotoxic T cells. These have proved to be either free tumour antigens released by the tumour or else complexes of these with antitumour antibody. In either case, the T cell is pre-empted from attacking the tumour cell itself.

Non-specific response to tumour cells

Natual killer (NK) cells are a heterogenous group of Fc receptor-bearing cells present in healthy subjects and have the morphology of large granular lymphocytes but are neither typical B nor T lymphocytes. In fact, there is some evidence to suggest a relationship to promonocytes. NK cells are cytotoxic *in vitro* to many, but by no means all, tumour cell lines. The susceptible tumour cells have one or more surface structures in common, recognizable by NK cells, which then bind to the tumour cell via corresponding receptors (Fig. 7.2e). This close cell apposition leads to tumour cell death by an as yet unspecified mechanism. The surface structures recognized by NK cells are not conventional tumour antigens and indeed may be shared by certain non-tumour cells.

Interferon certainly has an effect against certain types of malignancy, for example osteosarcoma, and interferon can directly inhibit the growth of the cancer cell and/or it can mediate its effect via NK cells. It increases the number and cytotoxicity of the NK cells.

Macrophages

These may constitute as much as 50 per cent of the population of inflammatory cells infiltrating a tumour. A marked histiocytic response in lymph nodes draining tumours such as carcinoma of the breast has been found to be a good prognostic feature. Besides their important role in processing antigen for recognition, macrophages are directly cytostatic or cytotoxic for certain tumour cell types. As for NK cells, the surface structures recognized are not conventional tumour antigens and it is likely that NK cells and macrophages recognize different structures. A number of substances can enhance the antitumour potential of macrophages including MIF, interferon and various bacterial preparations (Fig. 7.2e). Macrophages kill tumour cells by an extracellular mechanism not involving phagocytosis. There is some controversy as to whether close macrophage–tumour cell contact is needed, although there is much more evidence for the involvement of a soluble mediator than in other forms of cytotoxicity.

Interferon

As mentioned earlier, interferon can inhibit cell growth. Some types of normal cell are affected, as are many but not all tumour cell types. In animal models, interferon has shown promise as an anti-neoplastic agent. A number of preliminary studies in humans were encouraging although, as in many areas of cancer research, the better controlled the study the less dramatic the result and the value of interferon in cancer therapy remains unconfirmed. The effects of interferon are species specific and, until recently, human interferon has been available only in small amounts and at high cost. Many groups have now succeeded in inserting the human interferon gene into *Esch. coli* and in the near future interferon should be much cheaper and more readily available from such sources.

Summary

Compared with the rare cases of spontaneous remissions of tumours or their metastases, the relentless spread of malignant disease is only too common. It is self evident that the host's immune response fails to eradicate tumours or halt their growth once they have reached a certain size.

Hewitt and colleagues (1976) pointed out that in spontaneously occurring tumours in mice, immunity never followed transplantation of tumour cells, unlike in the virally or chemically induced neoplasms of the experimental immunologist.

Lately, some have even questioned Burnet's hypothesis that immune surveillance is constantly in operation in health, destroying malignant cells as they arise by spontaneous mutations. More recent evidence suggests that such spontaneous mutations are rather rare. Spontaneous tumours appear to be rare in immunologically privileged sites such as the hamster cheek pouch.

Non-immunological defences against cancer have been defined which could be more important than the immune system. For example, chemical carcinogens owe their mutagenicity to their ability to bind to the DNA in the host cell nucleus. Enzymatic mechanisms are available which are responsible for excision of the abnormal DNA sequences, which may arise in the normal subject. In xeroderma pigmentosum, there is an inherited tendency to develop skin cancers on surfaces exposed to sunlight. In these patients there is a genetically determined inability to repair ultraviolet-induced faults in the DNA of the skin cells; the appropriate enzymes are lacking.

Specific immunotherapy of cancer

If we accept that the immune response to tumours in humans is usually weak and ineffective, can it be artificially boosted by vaccination with the tumour cells? Mathé (1969) obtained a significant benefit for patients with acute lymphoblastic leukaemia by immunizing them with killed autologous leucocytes injected subcutaneously, combined with conventional chemotherapy. Subsequent studies have largely failed to confirm his results.

The immunotherapy of solid tumours has similarly been rather disappointing. Some success has been achieved with non-specific immunostimulants, such as the intrapleural instillation of BCG which resulted in a highly significant increase in survival rate and reduction in local tumour recurrence in patients undergoing excision of bronchogenic carcinoma. Similarly, a synthetic polyribonucleotide employed as an adjuvant to surgery and radiotherapy for malignant tumours resulted in an improved survival and reduced rate of local recurrences in patients with breast cancer. It is interesting that the same synthetic adjuvant can prevent spontaneous mammary tumours in mice.

It is still too early to say whether immunotherapy will become part of our armamentarium for the treatment of cancer. Until the tumour antigens are clearly defined and the cellular and humoral components of the immune response thoroughly understood, vaccination for the prevention of tumours remains a pipe dream. The new method for the large-scale production of monoclonal antibodies by mouse hybridomas could be very fruitful in this respect. It should be possible not only to define tumour antigens in this way, but also large amounts of this tumour-specific antibody might be linked to a radioactive isotope or a cytotoxic drug, and used for treatment of the malignancy. For diagnostic purposes, pulmonary metastases of choriocarcinomas producing human chorionic gonadotrophin (HCG) have been detected by use of [131]iodine-labelled antibody to HCG.

Oral premalignant states and oral cancer

In some dysplastic keratoses and in apparently all squamous cell carcinomas, there is a loss of ABO (H) antigens usually present on the cell surfaces of normal epithelium, conversely, actin antigens become detectable in the cytoplasm. These antigenic markers could be useful in distinguishing between benign and potentially malignant lesions of the oral epithelium. In advanced oral cancer, in common with malignancies arising at other sites, there is an impairment of cell-mediated immunity *in vivo* as assessed by skin testing with antigens such as dinitrochlorobenzene (DNCB).

Consistent with this, *in vitro* tests of cellular immunity have revealed that lymphocyte stimulation by mitogens is also impaired.

Blood lymphocytes from patients with early stage oral squamous cell carcinoma are significantly more cytotoxic for target cell lines derived from an oral cancer than are lymphocytes from control subjects, patients with advanced cancers have impaired lymphocyte cytotoxicity. In patients with early stage tumours, T lymphocytes with Fc receptors and NK cells contributed to this tumouricidal effect, whereas only NK cells were cytotoxic in control subjects or patients with advanced cancer. At the present time, interferon is being assessed as an agent in the treatment of oral cancer.

The Epstein–Barr virus: its association with Burkitt's lymphoma, infectious mononucleosis and nasopharyngeal carcinoma

In 1958, Burkitt described an unusual malignant lymphoma in children in East Africa. The jaws were commonly involved and the kidneys, ovaries, testes, spleen and lymph nodes were other sites of election.

Burkitt also noticed that the distribution of the tumour in Africa was determined by temperature and rainfall and suggested that this dependence on climatic conditions implied that an oncogenic virus was involved, and that this agent could be transmitted by an arthropod vector. This latter view is not now accepted, as discussed below.

Epstein and Barr subsequently identified viral particles in electron microscopic examination of lymphoblasts cultured from biopsies of Burkitt's lymphoma from African patients (Epstein *et al.* 1964). This Epstein–Barr virus (EBV) has proved to be a herpes virus and its viral DNA and EBV-associated nuclear antigens can be detected in Burkitt's lymphoma cells. Patients with Burkitt's lymphoma have significantly elevated antibody titres to some of the antigens of the virus. In a recent prospective study in Uganda, children found to have exceptionally high levels of serum antibody to EBV nuclear antigen in an initial survey went on to develop Burkitt's lymphoma far more frequently than those with low antibody titres.

Further evidence of the oncogenic potential of the EBV has come from experimental infection of owl monkeys and cottontop marmosets which was followed by malignant lymphomas. In the laboratory, infection of human B lymphocytes which have receptors for EB virus results in a continuously growing cell line ('immortalized'). An abnormal chromosome, No. 14, the result of an 8/14 translocation, has also been discovered in most cultures of Burkitt's lymphoma.

The natural history of Epstein–Barr virus infections

The link between infectious mononucleosis and the EBV was discovered fortuitously when a technician working with the virus developed infectious mononucleosis (glandular fever) and was found to have developed an elevated titre of specific EBV antibody. The primary infection by the EBV usually occurs in childhood. The virus is transmitted by kissing or by airborne droplets and enters the lymphoid tissue of the oropharynx, infecting B lymphocytes which have receptors for the virus. Memory lymphocytes and specific antibody are produced in response to the virus, conferring immunity. This primary infection in childhood is invariably asymptomatic (Fig. 7.3a). Thereafter, the individual sheds the virus into the oropharynx continuously throughout life.

In affluent societies, the primary infection may be delayed until late adolescence and in 50 per cent of cases there is an associated infectious mononucleosis. In this illness there is an exuberant proliferation of T lymphocytes responding to the EBV antigens on the surface of the B lymphocytes. Multiplication of T lymphocytes in the lymph nodes and spleen is responsible for the clinical enlargement characteristic of this condition, and T lymphoblasts spill over into the peripheral blood, forming the abnormal mononuclear cells which are a diagnostic feature (Fig. 7.3b).

In Burkitt's lymphoma, this multiplication of EBV-infected B lymphocytes is uncontrolled and a specific cytogenetic defect, the 14q+ marker chromosome, is present and a malignant lymphoma ensues.

Since the EBV has a worldwide distribution, the question arises as to why Burkitt's lymphoma is virtually confined to East Africa and Papua New Guinea? For the EBV to exert its oncogenic effect, it seems that the host must also have malaria, and it is not now thought that the oncogenic virus is transmitted by an arthropod vector. Burkitt's lymphoma may arise in these children because of an acquired immunodeficiency due to their concurrent malaria. As a result, the EBV-induced polyclonal proliferation of B lymphocytes in the primary infection becomes uncontrolled and a monoclonal tumour results (Fig. 7.3c).

Relevant to this concept, some recipients of renal transplants who have been given immunosuppressive therapy develop significant rises

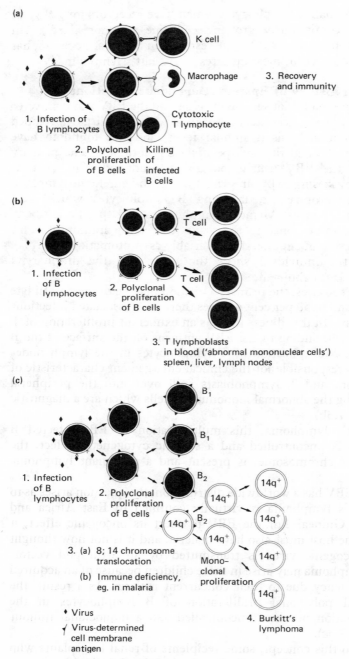

(a)

K cell

Macrophage

3. Recovery
and immunity

Cytotoxic
T lymphocyte

1. Infection of
B lymphocyte

2. Polyclonal   Killing
   proliferation of
   of B cells   infected
                   B cells

(b)

T cell

T cell

1. Infection
   of B
   lymphocytes

2. Polyclonal
   proliferation
   of B cells

3. T lymphoblasts
   in blood ('abnormal mononuclear cells')
   spleen, liver, lymph nodes

(c)

B₁

B₁

B₂

14q⁺

14q⁺

14q⁺

1. Infection
   of B
   lymphocytes

2. Polyclonal
   proliferation
   of B cells

14q⁺

14q⁺

14q⁺

14q⁺

Mono-
clonal
proliferation

14q⁺

3. (a) 8; 14 chromosome
       translocation

   (b) Immune deficiency,
       eg. in malaria

◆ Virus

↲ Virus-determined
  cell membrane
  antigen

4. Burkitt's
   lymphoma

Fig. 7.3 Possible results of Epstein–Barr virus infection. **(a)** Normal asymptomatic infection. **(b)** Infectious mononucleosis. **(c)** Burkitt's lymphoma.

in titre of serum antibody to the EBV. Immunosuppressive therapy also predisposes a patient to malignant lymphoma and, recently, EBV-associated nuclear antigens and viral antigens have been identified in some lymphomas occurring in immunosuppressed states.

Alternatively, it is possible that Burkitt's lymphomas represent a malignant proliferation of the clone of B lymphocytes arising from a single somatic mutation occurring during cell division in response to infection by both malaria and the EBV. Vaccination against malaria, or its eradication by present-day conventional methods, seems a logical approach to the long-term prevention of Burkitt's lymphoma.

Nasopharyngeal carcinoma

The Epstein–Barr virus has also been implicated in the aetiology of this squamous cell carcinoma of the nasopharynx which characteristically features a dense lymphocytic infiltrate. Patients with nasopharyngeal carcinoma were found to have significantly raised titres of antibody to the EBV, whereas patients with cancer of the lips or the oral cavity proper had low titres or were seronegative. The EBV–DNA genome has been detected in the nucleic acid of tumour cells. The fact that it is the commonest tumour in southern Chinese men and the second commonest in women of this race suggests that susceptibility to nasopharyngeal carcinoma is genetically determined.

Besides this inherited tendency, environmental factors may also play a part in the pathogenesis of nasopharyngeal carcinomas, according to epidemiological evidence. Surveys have established that, whereas southern Chinese immigrants to the United States of America and Australia have the same high incidence of nasopharyngeal carcinoma as in China, their descendants born in these western countries develop the tumour less frequently, although the incidence remains above that of Australian and American citizens of Caucasian origin.

References

Burkitt, D. (1958). A sarcoma involving the jaws in African children. *British Journal of Surgery* **46**, 218–23.

Burnet, F. M. (1965). Somatic mutation and chronic disease. *British Medical Journal* **1**, 338–42.

Epstein, M. A., Achong, B. G. and Barr, Y. M. (1964). Virus particles in cultured lymphoblasts from Burkitt's lymphoma. *Lancet* **i**, 702–703.

Hewitt, H. B., Blake, E. R. and Walder, A. S. (1976). A critique for active host defence based on personal studies of 27 murine tumours of spontaneous origin. *British Journal of Cancer* **33**, 241–59.

Mathé, G. (1969). Approaches to the immunological treatment of cancer in man. *British Medical Journal* **iv**, 7–10.

Further reading

Immunity and neoplasia

Catalona, W. J., Sample, W. F. and Chretien, P. B. (1973). Lymphocyte reactivity in the cancer patient: correlation with tumour histology and clinical stage. *Cancer* **31**, 65–71.

Currie, G. A. (1979). *Cancer and the Immune Response*, 2nd edn. Edward Arnold, London.

Dabelsteen, E. and Fulling, H. J. (1971). A preliminary study of blood group substances A and B in oral epithelium exhibiting atypia. *Scandinavian Journal of Dental Research* **79**, 387–93.

Fujibayashi, T., Sato, O. and Itoh, H. (1979). Stage-related, cell-mediated cytotoxicity with effector cell analysis and computation of cytotoxicity of T cells and non-T cells. *Cellular Immunology* **44**, 225–41.

Heberman, R. B. and Holden, H. T. (1978). Natural cell-mediated immunity to tumours. *Advances in Cancer Research* **27**, 305–377.

Roberts, J. J. (1980). Carcinogen-induced DNA damage and its repair. *British Medical Bulletin* **35**, 25–31.

Wanebo, H. J., Jun, M. Y., Strong, E. W. and Oettgen, H. (1975). T cell deficiency in patients with squamous cell cancer of the head and neck. *American Journal of Surgery* **130**, 445–51.

Epstein–Barr virus infections

Burkitt, D. P. and Wright, D. H. (1970). *Burkitt's lymphoma*. E. & S. Livingstone, Edinburgh and London.

Epstein, M. A. (1978). Epstein–Barr virus—discovery, properties and relationship to nasopharyngeal carcinoma. *I.A.R.C. Scientific Publications* **20**, 333–45.

Klein, G. (1977). Epstein–Barr virus, infectious mononucleosis and naso-pharyngeal carcinoma. *Israeli Journal of Medical Science* **13**, 716–24.

Köhler, G. and Milstein, C. (1975). Continuous cultures of fused cells secreting antibody of predefined specificity. *Nature* **256**, 495–7.

Purtilo, D. T. (1980). Epstein–Barr virus-induced oncogenesis in immunodeficient individuals. *Lancet* **i**, 300–303.

8

Immunodeficiency

Defects of the specific and non-specific aspects of the immune system are of particular significance for two reasons. Firstly, the oral and dental manifestations of immunodeficiency may be difficult to treat. Secondly, the incidence and severity of oral and dental disease may indicate the part played by the immunodeficiency in contributing to or protecting against those diseases.

Immunodeficiency (ID) may be primary, due to congenital defects in the immune system, or secondary, arising from diseases or drugs which affect the lymphoid system. Either the cellular or antibody-producing components of the immune system, or both, may be affected (Table 8.1).

Primary or congenital immunodeficiency

Defective specific immunity

An example of such an ID is severe combined immunodeficiency. The thymus is very small and the lymphoid tissues of the appendix and Peyer's patches are absent; there is susceptibility to bacterial, viral and fungal infections and, unless maintained in a germ-free environment, the patients die within two years of birth. In this disease, both antibody and cell-mediated immune reactions are profoundly depressed.

Virtually complete absence of humoral defence mechanisms is found in X-linked hypogammaglobulinaemia (serum IgG 1/10 of normal, serum IgA and IgM 1/100 of normal) although cell-mediated responses are normal. The disease has an X-linked recessive pattern of inheritance and boys with the disease are susceptible to pyogenic infections. Partial defects in immunoglobulin synthesis may affect IgG, IgA and IgM serum levels, and radial immunodiffusion (see Fig. 1.6) is one of the techniques used to detect deficiencies of individual immunoglobulins. In the Di George syndrome the lack of a thymus leads to a deficiency of cell-mediated immunity and is also associated with absence of the parathyroid glands and abnormalities of the great

Table 8.1   Some examples of immunodeficiency states

	Congenital or primary		Acquired or secondary	
Specific		Non-specific	Specific	Non-specific
T cell		Phagocytosis complement	Hodgkins disease, leukaemia, lymphosarcoma, multiple myeloma, protein-losing renal disease, or gut disease, cytotoxic therapy, irradiation, corticosteroids	Cytotoxic therapy, irradiation
Di George syndrome				
B cell				
Hypogammaglobulinaemia				
Partial Ig deficiency				
(a) IgG ↓ or IgA ↓ IgM↑				
(b) IgA ↓ + IgM ↓ IgG normal				
(c) Either IgA ↓ IgM ↓ or IgG ↓				
Combined T + B cell				
Severe combined immunodeficiency				
Common variable hypogammaglobulinaemia				
Wiskott–Aldrich syndrome				

vessels. There is a normal level of circulating antibody; the children are extremely susceptible to viral infection but not to malignancies.

All the above are very uncommon. Other less well-defined entities involving defects in antibody and/or cell-mediated immunity are more common and these are classed as common variable hypogamma-globulinaemia. The commonest immunodeficiency disease is IgA deficiency, which affects about 1/700 of the population in the United Kingdom. Antibodies of the IgA class protect the mucosal surfaces and deficiencies lead to recurrent upper respiratory tract infection. About half of the IgA-deficient patients have problems with infection and it is possible that the other half do not because they compensate by an increase in the amount of secretory IgM which they produce. Although there is this tendency to increased upper respiratory tract infection, such children actually experience less gingival inflammation. They may be more susceptible to caries but this impression is based on initial information only. From the point of view of the aetiology of gingival disease, the reduced level of gingival disease in patients with IgA deficiency would support the suggestion that the patient's immune response in some way contributes towards the progress of the disease. It should be emphasized however, that gingival inflammation, although reduced, is still present; perhaps confirmation of the direct damaging effect of dental bacterial plaque.

Defective non-specific immunity

Defective phagocytes

This may take several forms. Congenital cyclical neutropenia is characterized by a periodic fall in the level of circulating neutrophil leucocytes, often accompanied by oral ulceration. Since the disease is cyclical, care should be taken in distinguishing it from true recurrent aphthous ulceration. Impaired chemotaxis occurs in the 'lazy leucocyte syndrome' (together with neutropenia) and Chediak–Higashi syndrome (together with neutropenia and impaired intracellular killing of bacteria). In general, neutropenia and agranulocytosis are accompanied by severe periodontal disease. In chronic granulomatous disease where phagocytosis proceeds normally but intracellular killing of the bacteria is impaired, approximately 1/5 of the patients suffer from ulcerative stomatitis. These 'phagocytic disorder' diseases offer support for the concept that neutrophils emigrating through the gingival crevice are of value in preventing the acute manifestations of periodontal disease and that poorly functional neutrophils may predispose to the more rapid progression of chronic periodontal disease. Indeed, patients suffering from idiopathic juvenile periodontitis have been shown to have neutrophils which have impaired chemotactic responses and which phagocytose poorly.

Complement defects

Primary deficiencies of complement are very rare. Secondary deficiencies may arise through disease in which rapid consumption of complement is occurring. C1 esterase-inhibitor deficiency (hereditary angio-oedema) is of dental relevance since the condition presents as periodical bouts of severe oedema, often affecting the mouth and pharynx, particularly after dental surgery.

Acquired immunodeficiency

Acquired ID may arise secondarily to disease of the lymphoid tissue such as Hodgkin's disease, multiple myeloma, leukaemia or lymphosarcoma. It may also be caused by protein loss due to renal or intestinal disease, by malnutrition and by infection, for example measles or malaria.

Treatment in the form of irradiation, cytotoxic drugs and corticosteroids may also depress lymphocyte reactivity and reduce antibody levels and cause neutropenia. In such patients, recurrent infections are common and are slow to respond to treatment. If teeth are present, a gingivitis or periodontitis may become florid, whereas if dentures are worn, minor abrasions readily ulcerate and overgrowth of candidal organisms may occur.

Further reading

Asherson, G. L. and Webster, A. D. B. (1980). *Diagnosis and Treatment of Immunodeficiency Diseases*. Blackwell Scientific, Oxford.

Index